Crack and Ice
Treating Smokable Stimulant Abuse

About the authors:

   Donald R. Wesson, M.D., is the Associate Research Director, Los Angeles Addiction Treatment Research Center; the Scientific Director at Merritt Peralta Institute Chemical Dependency Recovery Hospital in Oakland, California; and Associate Clinical Professor, Department of Psychiatry at the University of California, San Francisco.

   David E. Smith, M.D., is the Founder and Medical Director of the Haight-Ashbury Free Clinics in San Francisco; Research Director at Merritt Peralta Institute Chemical Dependency Recovery Hospital in Oakland, California; and Associate Clinical Professor of Occupational Medicine and Clinical Toxicology at the University of California, San Francisco.

   Susan C. Steffens, M.A., is the Research Coordinator at Merritt Peralta Institute Chemical Dependency Recovery Hospital in Oakland, California.

Crack and Ice
Treating Smokable Stimulant Abuse

Donald R. Wesson, M.D.
David E. Smith, M.D.
Susan C. Steffens

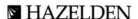 HAZELDEN

Hazelden Educational Materials
Center City, Minnesota 55012-0176

ISBN: 0-89486-822-5

Editor's Note:
   Hazelden Educational Materials offers a variety of information
on chemical dependency and related areas. Our publications do not
necessarily represent Hazelden's programs, nor do they officially
speak for any Twelve Step organization.

CONTENTS

Chapter

Chapter

Chapter

Chapter

TABLE AND FIGURES

ACKNOWLEDGMENTS

The authors gratefully acknowledge the assistance of friends and colleagues who critically reviewed successive drafts of the manuscript and made numerous helpful suggestions and comments, many of which we incorporated into the manuscript. In Oakland, staff at Merritt Peralta Institute Chemical Dependency Recovery Hospital were generous with their time and insights: Bill Wilson, the Executive Director; Barbara Stern; Rich Pelletier; the counselors; and most especially, Dr. Peter Washburn, the Medical Director. In Los Angeles, both Dr. Walter Ling, the Director of the Los Angeles Addiction Treatment Research Center, and Dr. Richard Rawson of Matrix, Inc., offered many constructive recommendations. Bill Chickering, our editor at Hazelden, made the manuscript much more readable through his thorough and cogent editing.

1
INTRODUCTION

Cocaine and methamphetamine are central nervous system stimulants: drugs that allay fatigue, enhance mental alertness, and elevate mood. Most societies sanction the use of mild stimulants such as caffeine and prohibit the use of strong stimulants such as amphetamine and cocaine. People who violate the prohibition are subject to criminal sanctions.

The social context of drug use and the way in which drugs are ingested have a great deal to do with the effects produced. For example, as part of their daily routine, many Indians in the Peruvian highlands chew coca leaves and drink tea that contains cocaine. Cocaine helps them work harder, reduces their fatigue, and elevates their mood. Their cocaine use enhances their work performance and increases their capacity for work.

The means of administering a drug is immensely important in determining its medical and social consequences. Peruvian Indians who *chew* coca leaves can do so for many years without ill effects. However, Indians in Lima and other urban centers in Peru who *smoke* coca paste suffer severe medical and psychiatric complications.[1]

COCAINE ABUSE

Before the Harrison Narcotic Act was passed in 1914, many patent medicines, alcoholic beverages, and cola drinks contained cocaine. There is no compelling evidence that cocaine, as a beverage, was abused, produced significant health risks, or caused significant social problems. Between 1914 and the early 1960s, intravenous heroin users were the primary consumers of cocaine. They injected cocaine, either by itself or by combining it with heroin. Some artists, writers, and musicians snorted cocaine, but cocaine use, in any form, was at that time clearly outside

1

mainstream culture. During those years, most Americans regarded cocaine use as deviant criminal behavior.

Attitudes toward cocaine as well as cocaine use patterns changed radically during the late 1960s and early 1970s, when a broad segment of American society began snorting cocaine. Consequently, many people came to view snorting cocaine in the same light as smoking marijuana: it was illegal, but most people did not consider its use serious criminal behavior. Many people who began using cocaine during this time did not use illicit drugs other than marijuana.

By the late 1970s, many middle- and upper-class people on the West Coast began smoking cocaine freebase. Most users bought cocaine hydrochloride in gram or greater quantities and made their own cocaine freebase using kits that were readily available at "head shops," through mail-order, and even in some gasoline service stations. The kits, which cost from fifteen to twenty dollars each, contained all the supplies needed to convert cocaine hydrochloride to cocaine freebase. The conversion process (described in detail in chapter 2) took several hours and required working with highly flammable ether.

Crack Cocaine

Also in the late 1970s, a new form of cocaine appeared: crack cocaine. Crack was not a new drug: it was freebase cocaine in another form (detailed in chapter 2). The use of crack cocaine first became popular in the Bahamas.[2] Shortly after that, crack smoking began on the East Coast of the United States.

In order to sell this new form of cocaine, dealers developed a new marketing strategy: they sold single ready-to-smoke "rocks" of crack at prices that ranged from five to twenty-five dollars each. This opened a new market for cocaine. Once available only to people with sizable incomes—or those willing to spend the time and take the risk of making freebase—cocaine had become accessible to lower-income working people, schoolchildren, and welfare recipients. Thus, the early 1980s saw a phenomenal increase in the new users of crack that attested to the dealers' effective marketing strategy.

By 1985, however, middle- and upper-income cocaine abusers were becoming disenchanted with cocaine. As the national media began to report deaths resulting from cocaine use and to print stories of addiction among sports figures and entertainers, cocaine—particularly crack—lost its illusion of safety. Once people realized they could die from using cocaine, its glamour waned, and many middle- and upper-income cocaine addicts sought treatment in private treatment programs. Among lower income groups and minorities (particularly Hispanics and Blacks) the number of cocaine users continued to increase, however.

Most major cities in the United States are now in the throes of the crack epidemic. City streets are no longer perceived as safe, and the increased costs of police, medical, and social services secondary to crack cocaine abuse are staggering. In San Francisco, for example, these costs are overwhelming,[3] and drug use tops the list of concerns for Bay Area residents.[4]

Some indicators suggest that the *peak* of the cocaine epidemic has passed. Statistics from the Federal Drug Abuse Warning Network and the National Household Survey suggest that cocaine use, including crack cocaine, is decreasing. Figure 1.1 on the following page, taken from a report of the National Institute on Drug Abuse, represents data from the Drug Abuse Warning Network, a reporting system of 405 hospital emergency rooms in twenty-one cities scattered throughout the country.[5]

The data show the total number of cocaine-related hospital emergency room admissions reported in the second quarter of each year from 1985 to 1990. The drop between 1989 and 1990 suggests decreasing cocaine use.

Although the number of new users appears to be decreasing, the need for treatment services continues to rise. Treatment of the currently addicted; the new users; and those with residual disability, including impaired "crack babies" born to addicted mothers, will continue to occupy medical and social service systems for many years to come. Unfortunately, service availability and accessibility

3

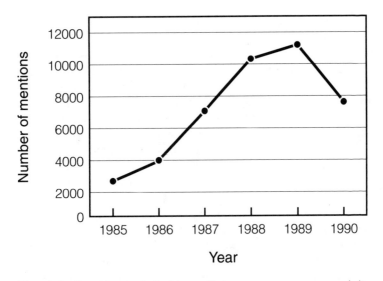

Fig. 1.1. Cocaine-related hospital emergency room visits

Cocaine-related hospital emergency room visits reported to the National Institute on Drug Abuse's (NIDA) Drug Abuse Warning Network. (The number of mentions are for the second quarter of each year.)

in the public sector is completely inadequate in all major cities in the United States.

Crime and Crack

Politicians and the media often use the crack epidemic to explain increasing crime statistics in major cities. For example, the lead article in the September 17, 1990, issue of *Time* magazine, bemoaning the "rotting of the Big Apple," notes an increase in crime of 25 percent in New York City since 1977 and suggests that the increase has been "fueled by the drug epidemic."[6] Territorial disputes among drug dealers, drug-induced paranoia in abusers, and crimes committed to obtain money to buy drugs—all contribute to increased crime. But while crack cocaine is clearly one contributor to growing crime statistics, other causes of crime are being neglected.

High rates of unemployment, racial tension, declining social services, a crumbling educational system, and alcohol abuse are also factors in the increased incidence of crime. So while drug abuse significantly contributes to urban crime and violence, drug abusers are also convenient scapegoats for the press and politicians. Politicians can safely acknowledge that the crack epidemic is out of control, point to force as the only way to control it, and ignore the pressing social problems that, in fact, prolong the crack epidemic. In spite of these deteriorating social conditions that increase the likelihood of crime, police services have been reduced in major cities across the country. For example, the New York City police force was 14 percent smaller in 1990 than it was in 1975.[7]

Meanwhile, guns have increasingly become part of the urban landscape, and people are increasingly willing to use them. In some areas, people are arming themselves in reaction to crack-related violence.

Even the crime directly related to crack will not necessarily disappear as the crack epidemic subsides. Some people predict that much of the violence will persist, particularly among the gangs that formed during the crack era.[8] The decline in crack use will mean a declining market for crack dealers; increased violence and gang wars may result as suppliers compete for the decreasing demand.

The Role of the Media in Cocaine Abuse

During the 1970s, the media glamorized the lifestyle of affluent drug dealers and the use of cocaine by celebrities. In effect, the media created an effective advertising campaign for cocaine and taught many people to view the drug as chic, exclusive, and daring. The media also distributed much misinformation.

Cocaine *Is* Addictive

The issue of addiction was confounded because professionals and lay people misunderstood the relationship between physical dependence and addiction. "Experts" often expressed the opinion that cocaine was not addictive. Their definition of addiction, however, used opiates or alcohol as a model. With either, there is marked tolerance, physical dependence, and an obvious withdrawal syndrome. On the one hand, the withdrawal syndrome from opiates and alcohol produced changes in blood pressure, pulse, temperature, and other easily measured physiological changes. On the other hand, cocaine withdrawal produced no obvious physiological changes. The effects were largely subjective: depressed mood, fatigue, irritability, and alterations in sleep patterns. Because of the absence of physical dependence, experts erroneously concluded that cocaine was not addictive.

Animal researchers further compounded the error. Because they could not observe physiological withdrawal symptoms in laboratory animals, they also concluded that cocaine was not addictive.

The "expert" opinion that cocaine was not addictive fostered cocaine's widespread acceptance during the 1970s. Many cocaine users who became addicted to cocaine were genuinely surprised.

By the early 1980s, it was apparent from the number of people in all socioeconomic classes whose lives had become dominated by the pursuit of cocaine that the drug was, in fact, addictive. The media focus shifted. Now drug researchers began to describe the intense euphoria produced by cocaine and the compulsive use patterns that people developed for the drug. Unlike the earlier research into cocaine withdrawal, there were good animal laboratory models for "compulsive use." Laboratory animals allowed to self-administer cocaine would continue to do so until they had seizures or died. Most people got the implied message. If animals would self-administer cocaine until they killed themselves, and people would use cocaine until they lost their families, jobs, and financial resources, cocaine must be an extremely powerful and reinforcing euphoriant.

The Appeal of Cocaine

While the addictive potential of cocaine deters many from use, the media publicity often piques the curiosity of others who are willing to risk becoming addicted to experience intense euphoria. For the dedicated pharmacological adventurer, addictive *potential* is not a deterrent from use. The danger of addiction, the illegality, and the high cost of cocaine add to its appeal. No one who begins to use cocaine believes he or she will develop medical complications or be the one to become addicted.

Another reason cocaine and cocaine freebase are appealing is the ways they can be used: by snorting and smoking. This appeals to users who buy the lie that you are not a real drug addict unless you stick a needle in your arm. And, in the era of AIDS, even the most adventuresome drug experimenter is reluctant to use a needle.

Smoking cocaine fit particularly well with the established behavior of the mainstream culture. The cigarette and the entertainment industries have acculturated people to view smoking cigarettes as glamorous, sexy, and a symbol of independence.

Treatment and Cocaine

Between 1980 and 1988, the number of cocaine addicts seeking treatment increased in both public and private drug treatment programs. Private physicians also treated greater numbers of patients for complications of cocaine abuse. For many reasons, that trend is heading downward. One reason is the widespread urine testing in the workplace. Another reason involves the cutbacks on insurance benefits covering treatment of addiction. Overall, demand for treatment in private programs is declining. At the same time, demand for treatment in public programs continues to increase.

Proprietary drug treatment programs have responded resourcefully and have devised treatment modalities specifically tailored to cocaine abuse. Some of these will be described in detail in chapter 5. They include cocaine recovery support groups, resort retreats, aversive therapy, short- and long-term residential treatment, and outpatient treatment services.

In spite of the availability of private treatment clinics and hospitals (many now advertise that they provide specific treatment for cocaine abuse), growing numbers of middle- and upper-income people are seeking treatment in alternative health care facilities such as the Haight-Ashbury Free Clinics, a San Francisco community-based health care and drug abuse treatment program. Many cocaine-dependent patients treated at the Haight-Ashbury clinics do not match the profile of patients treated in public sector clinics. Many are white, middle-class, employed, and have had no previous drug treatment.

People seek drug treatment in such clinics for a variety of reasons. Some are fearful that treatment in a private treatment program or by a private physician will alert their employer to their drug problem, because medical services are billed to insurance policies that are often through their employer.

An increasing number of crack-dependent, lower socioeconomic Hispanics and Blacks seek drug abuse treatment in community clinics because they cannot afford private treatment. With increased urine testing in the workplace, cocaine abusers who are dependent either quit their jobs because they know it is only a matter of time until their drug use will be discovered, or they are eventually fired. Even those who are still employed may have lost insurance benefits for private drug treatment. The crack epidemic coincided with increasing restrictions on private health benefits of all types, particularly for psychiatric and drug abuse treatment. As a result, public drug abuse programs are being overwhelmed with requests for services, while many private treatment programs are operating at less than half their capacity.

METHAMPHETAMINE ABUSE

In the early 1960s, methamphetamine was widely used to treat obesity, narcolepsy, and hyperkinetic behavior in children. It was available from pharmaceutical companies in pills or capsules and in an injectable form under the trade name of Methedrine.

Methamphetamine was also available from illegal laboratories.

The illicit methamphetamine, generally distributed as small crystals, was commonly called "crank." Addicts snorted it or dissolved it in water and then injected it.

In 1969 and the early 1970s, an epidemic of methamphetamine abuse occurred on the West Coast.[9] A few San Francisco physicians heightened interest in methamphetamine among intravenous heroin abusers by "treating" them with Methedrine. Subsequently, many heroin addicts began injecting Methedrine as a primary drug of abuse, obtaining it either by scamming physicians to get a prescription for Methedrine or by stealing the ampules.[10] Because of its abuse, the Drug Enforcement Administration (DEA) requested the pharmaceutical company that manufactured Methedrine to withdraw it from the market. This had little effect on the abuse of methamphetamine by intravenous drug abusers because the illicit production of methamphetamine (crank) rapidly increased.

In certain areas, such as the Haight-Ashbury district of San Francisco, this methamphetamine, or "speed," epidemic contributed greatly to the spread of viral infections such as hepatitis as a result of sharing dirty needles, and caused a surge in drug-related violence both as a result of stimulant paranoia induced by the drug and as a result of drug dealing.

In 1968, the Haight-Ashbury Free Clinics coined the phrase "Speed Kills" and mounted a public health campaign to educate people about the dangers of the drug. This speed epidemic had many of the same characteristics of the crack epidemic that followed in later years.

Ice

In the mid-1980s, "ice," a smokable form of methamphetamine, began to appear in the Philippines, Japan, and Hawaii. The United States DEA first seized quantities of ice in Hawaii during 1985. In 1990, the DEA seized ice in California that was apparently produced there.

Ice received so much media attention in 1990 that many addiction specialists were concerned the attention itself might help produce an epidemic of methamphetamine use. Without question, media attention has stimulated interest. The following conversation between two young men was overheard at a fast-food restaurant in San Francisco:

> *First man to his friend*: "Hey man, did you see that piece in the paper this morning about smoking ice? You know, on the front page."
>
> *His friend*: "Yeah, I definitely gotta try some of that."

For drug addicts and drug experimenters, the media is a valuable directory to the availability of new drugs and to potential sources of supply. The following lead paragraph from the *Los Angeles Times* illustrates the point.

> As the cars stream into the parking lot of the Towne Center mini-mall in Hollywood, "Ray" and the other drug dealers keep a wary eye out for customers and cops. . . . The exchange of crack cocaine for money was barely noticeable.[11]

The article showed a photograph of Towne Center and gave the cross streets. On the outside chance that anyone in Los Angeles was previously unable to locate a place to buy crack, they now knew where to go.

While the media may be responsible for educating people about the hazards of drug use, the sensationalized attention to drugs has probably done more to increase drug use than to decrease it.

Smokable forms of methamphetamine are potentially very toxic and can spread rapidly within a population. In January 1992, one of the authors, Dr. David Smith, visited addiction treatment facilities in Manila, the Philippines. There, ice is called "shabu." There are approximately 400,000 shabu addicts in the Philippines. The daily dose ranges from one to three grams per day, with shabu costing about ten to twenty dollars per gram, substantially less than cocaine. The shabu addicts combine large doses of benzodi-azepines, alcohol, and marijuana with the methamphetamine, creating a catastrophic polydrug abuse problem.

10

Ice as a Competitor of Crack

Cost and availability are major variables that control the spread of a drug epidemic. If ice in the United States became more available at a lower cost, then it would have the potential for wider use. However, since ice is a potential competitor for crack in certain East Coast cities, crack dealers fight turf battles to keep ice out of their area. In the United States, crack cocaine started on the East Coast and moved west; ice, emanating from Asia, hit Hawaii and the West Coast first and is now starting to spread east. As of mid-1992, ice use had not become epidemic in the United States, but the potential remains.

DRUG-FREE WORKPLACE INITIATIVES

The federal government has spurred major initiatives to encourage employers to discourage drug use among employees. As implemented, drug-free workplace programs rely heavily on involuntary pre-employment and employee urine testing. These programs have stimulated lively debates among professionals and are still controversial.

Anecdotal evidence suggests that testing decreases drug use among casual users and may result in some heavy users obtaining drug abuse treatment. But the decrease of drug-using employees has been accomplished primarily through attrition rather than through rehabilitation. Employers often fire employees when their drug use is detected.

Therapeutic Uses of Drug Testing

The arguments against involuntary urine drug testing for management purposes should not be extended to the therapeutic uses of urine drug testing in a drug abuse treatment context. Here, drug testing serves the purposes of preventing slips, detecting relapse, monitoring medication compliance, preventing contamination of the therapeutic environment, clarifying diagnosis, and ensuring a safe return to the workplace.

To prevent slips: Patients who know that their drug use will be detected have additional incentive to remain abstinent. Since cocaine metabolites and methamphetamine are detectable in urine for three to five days following a single use, random testing once or twice weekly will capture most slips from abstinence.

To detect relapse: The acknowledged purpose of testing is to detect relapse early so that appropriate clinical intervention (such as escalation of treatment intensity or hospitalization) can be made before the patient's drug use spins out of control. Patients who slip from abstinence often try to keep the slip a secret because they fear loss of privileges, are embarrassed, or don't want to disappoint their counselor, spouse, or employer. Patients may deny the seriousness of the slip and believe that they can stop their drug use on their own and no one will be the wiser. In this way, drug testing can cut through patients' denial.

To monitor compliance with therapeutic medications: The purpose is to verify that patients are actually taking the medications prescribed, such as methadone. From the program's perspective (as well as regulatory agencies), this form of monitoring is intended to decrease diversion of therapeutic medications. Methadone-maintained patients whose urine tests negative for methadone may be diverting their methadone to others.

To prevent drug contamination of the therapeutic environment: The purpose is to detect (and get rid of) "bad apples" who may undermine other patients' sobriety. The therapeutic environment must be protected from residents who are surreptitiously using drugs and who may recruit other patients in the program to join them in drug use.

To clarify medical and psychiatric diagnosis: The purpose of testing is to distinguish drug-induced disorders from those not produced by drugs (such as distinguishing paranoid schizophrenia from amphetamine-induced psychosis).

To ensure a safe return to the workplace during treatment: The purpose is to assure the employer, medical board, and so on that the patient is abstinent from drugs and can continue to work while undergoing treatment.

THE LANGUAGE OF ADDICTION

Language shapes our thinking, especially when it comes to the topic of drug addiction. We can speak of a drug use episode after treatment as a "relapse," or a "treatment failure." The choice of words influences our perception. The drug abuse field is also rich in metaphorical language, such as the *war* on drugs, the *journey* of recovery, a *detour* from abstinence, or the *disease* of chemical dependency. They can be powerful communication tools because they express ideas and often evoke subconscious beliefs and powerful emotions.

Many controversies in the substance abuse treatment field come from a misuse or misunderstanding of metaphors. A metaphor is an analogy, and the analogy is never precise. The use of a metaphor is fraught with danger if the person using it insists on its Truth. A metaphor can blind its user to alternative ways of thinking and introduce distortions that are difficult to perceive.

The Disease Metaphor

The hotly debated controversy about the disease model of drug abuse illustrates the point. Some insist that drug abuse *is* a chronic disease analogous to diabetes. The problem, of course, is that *unlike* diabetes, the biochemical abnormalities that *cause* drug abuse are unknown. Those who insist on the veracity of the disease model assert that it is only a matter of time until researchers unravel the biochemical or chromosomal basis of drug abuse. Proponents stress that the exact biochemical basis does not have to be understood before a pathological state with characteristic signs and symptoms can be defined as a disease. For example, it wasn't until the twentieth century that the biochemical basis of diabetes was understood, but those who argue against the disease model assert that it has not been proven and that alternative models, such as social learning, explain as much about people's drug abuse as does the disease model.

Although organizations such as the American Medical Association (AMA) have declared that all drug dependency, including alcoholism, is a disease, the issue remains controversial. The usefulness of the disease metaphor in working with drug abusers does not depend on its scientific validity. In other words, we can think of drug abuse and "treat" it as *though* it were a disease.

The disease metaphor has different meanings when used in the context of Twelve Step recovery or by physicians who are not addiction specialists. Within the Twelve Step context, viewing drug abuse as a chronic, progressive disease reduces the guilt and self-loathing of people who have "hit bottom." Although physicians don't object to using the disease model for the purpose of reducing guilt and self-loathing, they generally consider the treatment of disease as their turf. This clashes with the Twelve Step definition of disease, because Twelve Step groups view drug abuse as a disease for which medical treatment is often not only unnecessary but generally contraindicated.

Addiction specialists find themselves in a dilemma because they must reconcile the differing views of two groups: their medical colleagues, and the patients they treat who are involved in Twelve Step recovery work.

The Medical Treatment Model of Drug Abuse

Much criticism of the disease model of drug abuse is based on a misunderstanding of the medical model of treatment. Many people argue that the disease model relieves the drug abuser of all responsibility. This is a common misunderstanding. A person who has a medical disease is not held at "fault" for having the disease; however, he or she must seek appropriate medical care, follow medical advice, and not do things that would complicate the condition. In other words, the person is not responsible for having a disease, but is responsible for his or her behavior during recovery from the disease.

Those who argue against medical treatment for addiction generally characterize the medical model of treating illness this way: Patients present their medical complaints to their physicians. The physicians, who view themselves as experts and who know best what their patients "need" in order to treat their illness, respond by prescribing medications. The patient's role is to accept the treatment prescribed and to follow the physician's orders.

The authoritative, omniscient physician interacting with a passive, recipient patient is a common mode of physician-patient interaction. It is an efficient and cost-effective way to treat most patients with short-term, time-limited illnesses for which a complete *cure* is likely. It is not, however, the only "medical model."

Critics of the Medical Model

Advocates of the recovery model of drug abuse treatment are critical of the "medical model" because the patient is passive, and only minimally involved in the healing process. The detractors of the "medical model" accurately perceive that this medical model is not effective for treatment of addiction. The treatment of addiction requires that patients be actively engaged in the healing process and that they take responsibility for much of the treatment.

Many physicians who treat chronic illnesses—for example, diabetes or chronic pain—encourage a collaborative relationship with their patients. In this "rehabilitation model," physicians educate patients about the illness and encourage patients' participation in support groups. In this case, the physician is a team leader and patient guide. The physician prescribes and coordinates therapies, assesses the extent of disability, helps patients access insurance and other disability benefits, and provides them with counsel about how to manage their illness and avoid medical complications. The physician-patient interaction has many parallels to the addiction treatment counselor, and many principles of the rehabilitation model and the recovery model are the same.

Psychotherapy Is Not the Medical Model

Psychotherapists do not use the passive medical model. All psychotherapy builds on the principle that healing occurs from the patient's actively participating in the process. Psychotherapy, whatever the theoretical orientation, also has an educational component. (In chapter 5, we will review the role of psychotherapy in the treatment of addiction.) The primary criticism of psychotherapy when used for the treatment of addiction is not its use of the medical model but its concept of addiction as a secondary symptom of an underlying psychopathology.

Medical Model of Addiction Medicine

Many physician addiction specialists do not use the medical model. Nor is it the basis for the kind of physician-patient interaction advocated by the American Society of Addiction Medicine (ASAM), although ASAM seeks to expand treatment of addictive disease within the context of mainstream medicine.

It would be more accurate to speak of the "medical models of treatment," each having strengths and weaknesses. The authoritative, physician-prescribed model is efficient and cost-effective for treating most short-term disorders. It is not appropriate for treating chronic illnesses such as drug addiction. In contrast, the rehabilitative model, which is costly in terms of physician time, has parallels to the chemical dependency counselor's role and is an effective model for managing many chronic illnesses, including drug abuse. The psychotherapeutic therapies are costly but may be of particular benefit for patients with combined psychiatric and addiction disorders.

Understanding the false dichotomy between a single "medical model" and the "recovery model" will enhance counselors' appropriate referral of their clients to medical treatment. In addition, it will improve communication between counselors and addiction medicine specialists.

Social Policy and the War Metaphor

Another example of metaphorical thinking that produces much difficulty is the war metaphor—the war against drugs. Federal and state governments choose the war metaphor to describe many large-scale social projects, such as the war on poverty. Choosing a war metaphor to apply to domestic social projects could be bureaucratic sloth, linguistic incompetence, or political expediency, but no government official who thought very deeply about its meaning would use the war metaphor. War is the last-ditch effort of a government of one country to exert its will over another country, an activity that sanctions the suspension of the rules of basic decency and ignores the sanctity of human life.

Sometimes the war metaphor is benign, such as *the war on cancer,* or *the war on poverty.* Here the targets are diseased tissue or an abstract construct. The *war on drug abuse*, however, is not benign because *people* are its targets (drug dealers and drug users), and the battlegrounds include United States cities. When it comes to drug abuse, however, the term is not simply a metaphor. The "war" on drugs is *thought about* in war terminology, and it has some aspects of *real* war. The dealers and narcotics agents are real combatants using high-tech weaponry. There are real casualties and innocent victims caught in the crossfire. Each year, thousands of people are terrorized, injured, or killed.

GRASS ROOTS THEORY ABOUT THE CRACK EPIDEMIC AND THE WAR ON DRUGS

In working with minority addicts and their families, counselors—particularly if they are not of the same racial or ethnic background as their clients—must understand minority beliefs and cultural backgrounds. Many within Black communities hold a certain theory about the government's role in stopping the crack epidemic. In its most complete form, the theory is that the government launched the "war" against illicit drugs not to reduce drug use but to politically justify the oppression of people who oppose its policies. In this view, the government's efforts at drug interdiction are only a symbolic gesture. Even drug enforcement officials acknowledge that government agents seize only a small portion of the drugs that come across the United States borders.

Minorities' Resistance to Treatment

Minority addicts can use this theory to subtly resist treatment. In order to overcome client resistance, counselors must be aware of the theory and be willing to discuss it openly. The counselor must also be willing to listen carefully to ideas that may contradict his or her world view. The correctness of the ideas cannot be challenged. Confrontation will alienate the addict, who may then feel justified in quitting or sabotaging treatment.

Many Black people, including those who do not use illicit drugs, hold that the government will continue to allow cocaine to enter the country as long as the primary consumers are Blacks and Hispanics. Some even maintain that the United States government actively participates in bringing cocaine into the country.

Further, many people (including crack addicts) claim that the government should, and could, provide treatment services, but that it withholds programs and suppresses new drug treatments because it wants the crack epidemic to continue within minority communities.

The conspiracy viewpoint is not confined to the Black community. Government response (or, more accurately, nonresponse) to the crack epidemic can be viewed as a facet of racism, since crack use and dealing are now largely centered in the Black communities in the mainland United States. Greil Marcus, a former editor of *Rolling Stone*, was quoted in an interview:

> I think that many of the people leading this country are perfectly happy to see the black communities around the country destroying themselves, to see the life expectancy of a young black man drop every year, and to have it be a fact that for black men between the ages of eighteen and thirty—I may not have the years exactly

right—murder is the number one cause of death. I think people are very happy with that.[12]

Although crack is distributed within the black community largely by Blacks, cocaine production and importation into the United States are neither instigated nor controlled by Blacks. As a result, Blacks claim to be victimized by cocaine. This view of Blacks as victims has made its way into popular culture. For example, director and writer John Singleton's movie *Boyz 'N the Hood* portrays the black community's experience of being victimized by non-black drug importers.

The Counselor's Role

To help minorities achieve recovery, drug counselors should not argue with clients about the correctness of the conspiracy theories, but rather help addicts change their self-concept from victim to being an active participant in recovery. The counselor should be nonjudgmental of the addict's beliefs, but try to understand how the beliefs developed in the context of the addict's background and environment.

Chapter 1
ENDNOTES

1. F. R. Jeri, C. Sanchez, and T. del Dozo, "The Syndrome of Coca Paste: Observations in a Group of Patients in the Lima Area," *Journal of Psychoactive Drugs* 10 (1978): 361-70.
2. J. F. Jekel et al., "Epidemic Freebase Cocaine Abuse—Case Study from the Bahamas," *Lancet* 1 (1986): 459-62.
3. B. Gordon, "Crack's Incredible Cost to San Francisco: City Could Go Broke Over Drug," *San Francisco Chronicle* (21 February 1989): 1.
4. R. G. McLeod, "Drugs, AIDS Top Bay Area Concerns," *San Francisco Chronicle* (3 March 1989).
5. K. H. Sobel, "Cocaine-Related Hospital Emergency Room Visits Drop 30 Percent," *NIDA Notes* 5 (1990): 6.

6. J. Attinger, "The Decline of New York," *Time* 136 (17 September 1990): 36-44.
7. Attinger, 36-44.
8. G. Gugliotta and M. Isikoff, "Violence in the '90s: Drugs' Deadly Residue," *Washington Post* 313 (Sunday, 14 October 1990): 1.
9. D. E. Smith and D. R. Wesson, *Uppers and Downers* (Englewood Cliffs, N. J.: Prentice-Hall, 1973).
10. Smith and Wesson, *Uppers and Downers.*
11. J. Meyer, "Flyers Advertise 24 Hour Drug Sales Outside Mini-mall," *Los Angeles Times* (1 March 1991): B7.
12. H. Benson, "Now We Are Engaged in a Great Cultural Civil War," *San Francisco Focus* 37 (December 1990): 145.

2
PHARMACOLOGY OF COCAINE
AND METHAMPHETAMINE

COCAINE

In the United States, cocaine is available in two forms:

1. the hydrochloride salt
2. the freebase

Pharmaceutical chemists call the freebase form "cocaine alkaloid." Cocaine hydrochloride dissolves in water and is the form of the drug that is snorted or injected. It is not commonly smoked. Cocaine hydrochloride has a high melting point (195 degrees centigrade) and vaporizes at a still higher temperature, so that much of the cocaine is destroyed in attempts to smoke it. Smoking is an inefficient way of using cocaine hydrochloride.

Crack is a freebase form of cocaine. This form does not dissolve in water, so it cannot be injected or snorted. It does, however, have a low melting point and vaporizes at a low temperature. Smoking is a very efficient way to use cocaine freebase. Figure 2.1 shows the chemical structure of cocaine freebase.

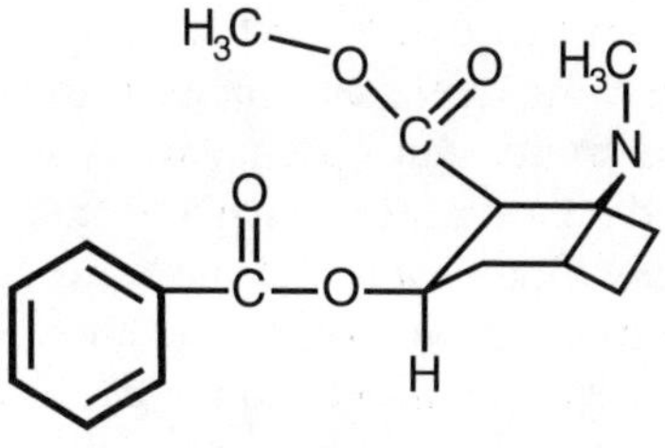

Cocaine

Fig. 2.1. Chemical structure of cocaine freebase

Preparation of Cocaine Freebase

The freebase form of cocaine can be produced in one of two ways:

1. the water method, using baking soda
2. the ether-extraction method

The Water Method

Cocaine hydrochloride is first mixed with baking soda. The mixed powder is dissolved in water, and the resulting solution is boiled. The baking soda (sodium bicarbonate) reacts with the cocaine hydrochloride to produce the cocaine freebase. Cocaine freebase melts just below the boiling point of water (100 degrees centigrade). Cocaine freebase is insoluble in water and slightly heavier. It forms little globs that settle at the bottom of the container. By gently swirling the container, the "cooker" causes the small globs to form a single liquid glob. As the water cools below the melting point of freebase (97 degrees centigrade), the cocaine freebase becomes a hard solid rock. (Before the advent of crack on the East Coast, freebase users on the West Coast referred to freebase prepared by the water method as "rock.")

The Ether-Extraction Method

The first step to making freebase by the ether extraction method is to dissolve the cocaine hydrochloride in a small amount of water. Then sodium or ammonium hydroxide is added to the solution. The sodium or ammonium hydroxide reacts with the cocaine hydrochloride to make cocaine freebase. Since the freebase is not soluble in water, it turns the solution an opaque milky white. In the second step, ether is poured on top of the water solution. (The ether is lighter than water and floats on top of the water like oil on vinegar.) The solutions are then mixed together. Since freebase cocaine is soluble in ether, it moves to the ether layer. The leftover sodium or ammonium hydroxide and any water-soluble "cuts" in the cocaine, such as lactose, remain in the water layer. After the solution sits for a moment, the ether layer (containing the freebase cocaine) floats to the top of the water. The ether layer is drawn off the top of the solution with an eye dropper and put on a dish. As the ether evaporates, small white crystals of cocaine freebase appear.

Until the early 1980s, freebase kits containing all the necessary chemicals (except, of course, cocaine hydrochloride) were available for mail-order purchase or were sold in drug paraphernalia shops. Drug paraphernalia laws have since made the sale of these kits illegal throughout the United States.

The end product, cocaine freebase, is chemically the same whether it's prepared by the water method or the ether method. The appearance of cocaine freebase varies widely, depending on how it has been prepared. Freebase prepared by the water method results in a hard, solid pellet that resembles a small white rock. Freebase prepared by the ether-extraction method results in small white crystals.

Street Names for Cocaine Freebase

Street terminology referring to cocaine freebase is confusing. Some people refer to any form of freebase cocaine as "crack"; others restrict the term "crack" to refer only to the solid "rock" form of cocaine freebase produced by the water method. Other street names for crack include "white dove" and "hubba."

SUBJECTIVE EFFECTS OF SMOKED COCAINE

The subjective effects of cocaine freebase vary considerably from person to person and may be different from one time to the next for the same person. The medical health and psychological makeup of the person, the social context, the amount the person smokes, and the period of time over which cocaine is smoked all influence the subjective effects.

The following story of a young woman in treatment for cocaine abuse illustrates several important points.

When I got home, my boyfriend and his friend were sitting huddled over in the middle of the living room floor, taking one hit after another. They were disgusting. The living room was a mess. There were loose pieces of aluminum foil scattered all over. For a long time they didn't even acknowledge that I had entered the room. Finally, my boyfriend asked if I wanted a hit.

Now, I've snorted a lot of coke, even shot it a few times. No big deal. While I made a straw from a piece of aluminum foil, my boyfriend held a piece of aluminum foil with a lighter underneath. The freebase melted and rolled around on the foil. I sucked up the smoke with the tinfoil straw. It was a good rush, but after one hit my pulse was pounding, and I had had enough. I got up and went to the kitchen to get something to eat. They stayed in the living room huddled like animals over the smoking aluminum foil—taking one hit after another. I couldn't see why they kept on doing it, hit after hit. They didn't quit until the base was all gone. By then, they were both paranoid, and they wanted me to give them some money so they could go get some more coke.

Over the next month, I did it with them a few more times like that. Then I joined them on the floor. I didn't stop until I came here.

This patient's story has elements that are commonly reported by other crack addicts in treatment. First, she snorted cocaine for some years without becoming addicted to it. Second, she was introduced to crack by her boyfriend, which is a way women commonly are introduced to crack. Although the subjective effects of smoking cocaine as opposed to snorting it were different, she didn't find the initial experience highly desirable. With repeated use, however, she rapidly lost control of her crack use and became obsessed with using it. Finally, she eloquently describes the total obsession addicts have with using cocaine once they begin smoking it.

Figure 2.2 illustrates some additional points regarding the subjective effects of smoking cocaine.

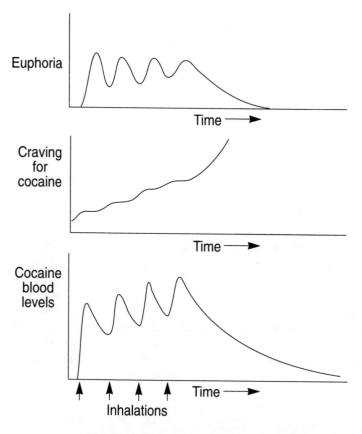

Fig. 2.2. Effects of cocaine smoking

This figure was developed after listening to many users in treatment describe their experience. Of particular importance is what happens with craving. Note that the craving increases soon after the user has taken a hit. It typically continues to escalate until the user has exhausted all means of acquiring more cocaine.

The first hit produces the most pleasurable subjective effect. Each subsequent inhalation produces less and less effect, though users keep trying to recapture the intensity of the first hit.

> The first hit was fantastic, but afterward, it was never the same. I kept taking more hits, trying to get the same effect as the first. I kept thinking I must be doing something wrong, like not inhaling deep enough, or not having the flame hot enough. Sometimes I would miss hits because I kept hearing noises behind me, and I would turn around to look. I know now that I was paranoid and was hallucinating, but at the time, the noises seemed real, and I had no idea that the cocaine was causing them.

PATTERNS OF COCAINE ABUSE

Snorting

By quickly inhaling through one nostril, a cocaine user vacuums cocaine hydrochloride onto the nasal mucosa. Being water-soluble, the cocaine hydrochloride is readily absorbed and enters the bloodstream. This is a reasonably efficient way of getting cocaine into the body, and a user can absorb lethal amounts of cocaine by inhaling, or "snorting," the drug.

The effects of the cocaine occur within minutes and may last several hours. The user obtains the stimulant effects, but not the "rush" of smoking or injecting cocaine.

Freebase cocaine cannot be snorted because it is not water-soluble.

Intravenous Injection of Cocaine

Since cocaine hydrochloride can be dissolved in water, a cocaine user can put the solution in a syringe and inject it. Before the mid-1970s, most intravenous abusers of cocaine were primarily heroin abusers who also abused cocaine alone or in combination with heroin (known as a "speedball"). In spite of the risk of HIV

26

infection and the availability of crack, intravenous cocaine abuse continues among the intravenous heroin abusers and former abusers who are on a methadone maintenance program.[1]

Smoking

Crack or cocaine freebase crystals are often smoked in glass pipes. Sometimes the pipes contain water, which cools the vapor with minimal loss of cocaine. The glass pipe has a bowl fitted on the bottom with one or more fine-mesh copper screens. The freebase is placed on the screen. The user heats the side of the bowl with a small butane torch or cigarette lighter. The freebase vaporizes into an aerosol, which is drawn into the lungs.

Smoking is an efficient way of getting cocaine to the brain. The cocaine enters the blood in the lungs just before that blood enters the left side of the heart. Within a few seconds, this blood reaches the brain. This method works faster than intravenous injection.

Cocaine freebase is sometimes put into a marijuana cigarette. A marijuana cigarette laced with crack is commonly called a "grimmie." Although smokers of grimmies are using crack, they view it as a less severe form of cocaine abuse than using a pipe. Some freebase abusers report using grimmies to control their cocaine use. When cocaine is smoked in marijuana, users report less compulsion for continued use and less difficulty sleeping after use.

The combination of crack cocaine and a tobacco cigarette is known as "caviar" (or "cavies") and, more recently, as "primmies." A cavie is prepared by grinding the crack to a powder and using the cigarette as a straw, sucking the cocaine into the cigarette. The advantage of a cavie is that it can be smoked in public without appearing that the person is smoking cocaine.

Some users will smoke cocaine hydrochloride in a tobacco or marijuana cigarette. This is inefficient because much of the cocaine hydrochloride is destroyed by the high temperature of the cigarette.

Some cocaine freebase abusers mix cocaine and freebase heroin together. The street term for smoking a mixture of cocaine and heroin is "chasing and basing."

COCAINE CRAVINGS

Cocaine cravings are the topic of frequent discussion among cocaine addicts and the people who treat them. In spite of the subjective intensity of cravings and their control of the addict's behavior, stimulant addicts have difficulty describing cravings. Addicts often describe them in terms of a "gut reaction." What is clear is that cocaine addicts episodically experience an intense and overpowering desire to use cocaine.

Cravings are usually environmentally triggered (such as by hearing a song, by seeing a picture of a crack pipe, or by being in a neighborhood) or are situationally triggered (for example, by meeting a friend with whom the addict has used cocaine or by seeing a dealer). One of the most common triggers patients report is payday: having money to spend. Cravings are intensified by access to cocaine and, once triggered, have a life of their own.

The addict experiences cocaine craving as an instinctual drive, such as that of hunger or the need to relieve sexual tension. Once the cocaine cravings are triggered, their relief becomes the addict's primary concern and may preempt drives such as hunger or sex. The addict believes that the cravings will be relieved by cocaine use and that, if not relieved, they will grow in intensity.

Much pharmacological treatment is directed toward *reducing the intensity* of craving for cocaine. Much psychosocial treatment is directed toward increasing the person's ability to *cope* with craving. The end goal for both types of treatment is to break the link between craving and drug-use behavior.

METHAMPHETAMINE

Figure 2.3 shows the chemical structure of methamphetamine.

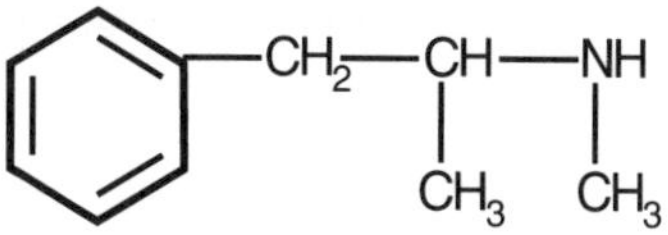

Methamphetamine

Fig. 2.3. Chemical structure of methamphetamine

Understanding the different forms of methamphetamine requires some knowledge of stereo chemistry. When a beam of polarized light passes through a liquid solution of some drugs, the molecules of the drug rotate the beam of light either to the right or to the left. If the rotation is to the right, it is called "dextro" rotary; if it is to the left, it is called "levo" rotary. This information is incorporated into the chemical name of a drug. The drug's name is prefaced by *d* (dextro) or *l* (levo) to indicate the direction in which the beam of light rotates.

The most common method of making illicit methamphetamine results in a product (dl-methamphetamine) in which half of the molecules of methamphetamine rotate the beam to the right; the other half rotate the beam to the left. The net result is no rotation.

The dextro and levo forms of methamphetamine have different physical properties and affect the brain differently.

Only the dextro-methamphetamine forms large crystals (under the appropriate conditions), while a mixture of the dextro- and · levo-methamphetamine forms small crystals about the size of salt. Methamphetamine users will sometimes claim they use "ice" (dextro-methamphetamine) when, in fact, they are using the dl-methamphetamine mixture. If they describe the methamphetamine as small crystals, it is most likely not ice.

Dextro-methamphetamine is many times more potent as a central nervous system stimulant than levo-methamphetamine.

Table 2.1 summarizes the forms of methamphetamine.

Table 2.1
Forms of Methamphetamine

Chemical Form	Common Generic or Street Name	Source
L-methamphetamine	Desoxyephedrine	Vicks Inhaler®
DL-methamphetamine HCL	Desoxyn®	Abbott Laboratories
	Crank	Illicit laboratories, U.S.
D-methamphetamine HCL	Ice	Illicit laboratories, U.S., Korea
methamphetamine freebase	Snott	Illicit laboratories

Ice

Ice is dextro-methamphetamine hydrochloride. The term "ice" refers to its appearance. Under appropriate conditions, it can crystallize into large crystals several inches long that are similar in appearance to quartz. The color ranges from none at all (clear) to yellow-brown. The process of making large ice crystals is the same as that of making rock candy. The d-methamphetamine is dissolved in warm water, and the water is allowed to cool slowly. The slower it cools, the larger the crystals.

Ice is water-soluble. If held between the thumb and forefinger, it will become slippery (like ice made from water) from the moisture on the fingertips.

Some people are under the impression that ice is the freebase form of methamphetamine. This is not true. Freebase methamphetamine is a liquid at room temperature.

Ice is also known as "crystal," "ice cream," "L.A. glass," "quartz," "rice," "batu," or "shabu." The term "crystal" can be confusing, since this is also the East Coast term used to refer to 4-methylaminorex (also called Euphoria or U4euH) and may also refer to PCP.

Ice smoking began in Asia and has since become common in Hawaii, where the distribution systems for both ice and cocaine freebase are the same. This contrasts with the mainland United States where street-level distribution of crack is primarily within the Black communities and street-level distribution of methamphetamine is primarily within white communities.

Crank

Until recently, all illicit synthesis of methamphetamine produced dl-methamphetamine hydrochloride. The crystalline form of methamphetamine, commonly called "crank," "crystal," or "speed," is still the most commonly produced form, although the DEA has raided a few illicit laboratories that were producing the *d* form of methamphetamine (ice).

The term "laboratories" is a misnomer. In California, most of the methamphetamine is made in the kitchens of private homes. The manufacture and distribution are largely controlled by the motor-cycle gang, Hells Angels. According to local California drug enforcement agencies, the Hells Angels contract with individuals to make the methamphetamine and supply the chemicals and the formula. After the methamphetamine is made, they buy the entire batch and distribute it to street-level dealers. By spreading the manufacturing over many small production units throughout California, they make the operation very difficult for drug enforcement officials to stop. Narcotic officers can bust the laboratories, but any individual laboratory is a small portion of the total production capacity.

The usual process for making methamphetamine involves the use of an organic solvent such as ether. Ether is highly flammable, and many houses involved in methamphetamine manufacturing have exploded and burned.

Licitly Produced Methamphetamine

Levo-methamphetamine, which causes little activity in the central nervous system, is an ingredient in Vicks Inhaler. Because l-methamphetamine has little central nervous system effect on mood, it is not a significant drug of abuse. Its importance to substance abuse is that it can produce a positive test for amphetamine in urine when the laboratory uses sensitive detection methods.[2]

Dl-methamphetamine is available as a prescription medication under the trade name Desoxyn. Physicians prescribe Desoxyn for treatment of hyperkinetic children and treatment of narcolepsy. In years past, it was also prescribed for weight control. However, current medical consensus is that the abuse potential of amphetamines such as Desoxyn exceed their potential benefits for weight control.

Methamphetamine can be smoked, injected, or snorted. Methamphetamine consumed by smoking is usually methamphetamine hydrochloride. It is usually smoked in small, straight glass pipes. It cannot be smoked in *water* pipes, as is cocaine freebase, because, unlike cocaine freebase, methamphetamine hydrochloride is water-soluble and would be trapped in the water. Some users place the methamphetamine powder on aluminum foil and hold a lighter under the foil in order to vaporize the methamphetamine. As with heroin, this mode of use is sometimes called "chasing the dragon."

As with cocaine, users can also put methamphetamine in a tobacco or marijuana cigarette and smoke it. However, methamphetamine freebase is liquid at room temperature, so some users dip cigarettes in the liquid in order to "smoke" it.

Subjective Effects of Smoked Ice

Users of ice who have also smoked crack generally report that initially, ice affects them less intensely and is less debilitating. Further, the effects of ice last much longer, and there is not the rapid craving for more, as with crack (see figure 2.4).

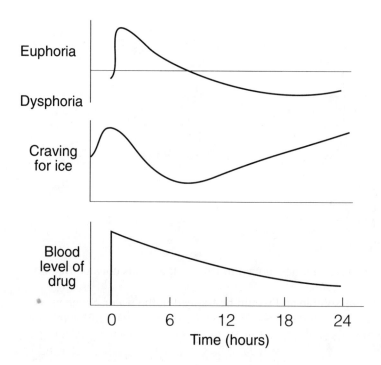

Figure 2.4. Effects of smoked ice

The difference in subjective effects between cocaine and methamphetamine is primarily due to differences in their rates of metabolism. Figure 2.5 illustrates this.

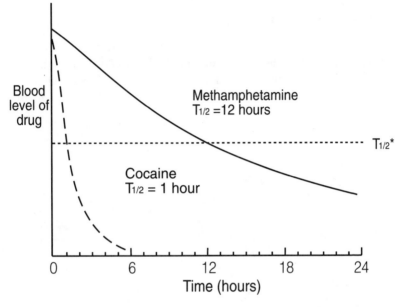

Fig. 2.5. Comparison of methamphetamine and cocaine metabolism

*Rates of drug metabolism are often compared in terms of their half-life; that is, the time required for the blood level to fall to one-half of its peak value.

DETECTION OF COCAINE AND METHAMPHETAMINE IN URINE

Both cocaine and methamphetamine are readily detected in urine specimens for several days following use. Urinalysis can be useful in identifying people who use crack or ice and in identifying relapse to drug use in patients who have been treated for drug dependency. The optimal use of urinalysis requires both a clinical sensitivity to the pitfalls of urinalysis and specific knowledge regarding the detection of cocaine and methamphetamine in urine.

Cocaine

Most urinalysis techniques do not detect cocaine itself, but cocaine's metabolite, benzoylecgonine. Both cocaine and benzoylecgonine are excreted in urine; however, cocaine disappears from the urine much more rapidly than benzoylecgonine. A urine sample will contain benzoylecgonine for two to five days following a single episode of cocaine use, and five to fourteen days following chronic use.

Urine screening techniques such as EMIT use a cutoff of 300 nanograms per milliliter of urine (sometimes expressed as 0.3 nanograms per liter). The cutoff value is the dividing line between a positive and a negative sample. If a urine specimen measures below the cutoff, it is reported as negative for cocaine; if it measures more than the cutoff, it is reported as positive for cocaine. It is important to be aware that the cutoff is not zero. The cutoff value is set by the equipment manufacturer to give as great a sensitivity as possible with as few false positives as possible. Setting the cutoff high has important consequences when monitoring patients. On the one hand, some patients may have used cocaine, but their urine values of benzoylecgonine will have dropped below the cutoff level and their urine results will be reported as negative. On the other hand, the cutoff is sufficiently high that patients are unlikely to test cocaine-positive from just being in the same room where cocaine is being used. Three hundred nanograms of benzoylecgonine in the urine indicates significant ingestion of cocaine.

The concentration of benzoylecgonine in urine is influenced by the amount of urine produced. The urine concentration of benzoylecgonine will be lowered if a patient drinks a lot of fluid before giving the urine sample. The fluid volume becomes important in samples whose values are near the cutoff value. Increasing fluid volume may result in diluting a sample below the cutoff value.

Methamphetamine

Methamphetamine is excreted unchanged in urine. Its excretion rate is highly dependent on the acidity or alkalinity of urine. The acidity or alkalinity of urine is usually expressed as its "pH value." A pH of 7 is neutral. Values less than 7 are acid; values greater than 7 are alkaline. The pH of urine normally varies between 6 and 8. As the urine becomes more acid, greater quantities of methamphetamine are excreted.

A common cutoff value for methamphetamine is 300 nanograms per milliliter. Because methamphetamine excretion is so influenced by urine pH as well as by urine volume, urinary values of methamphetamine are subject to much more variation than cocaine.

Some techniques for detecting methamphetamine in urine can confuse methamphetamine with phenylpropanolamine, which is a common ingredient in cough-cold medicines and diet aids and can be purchased in drug stores without a prescription. Phenylpropanolamine is also an ingredient in some prescription medications. There are, however, confirmation techniques that a urinalysis laboratory can use to distinguish methamphetamine from phenylpropanolamine.

Laboratory tests for methamphetamine do not distinguish between the dextro and levo isomers. L-amphetamine can be ingested in over-the-counter nasal inhalers used as nasal decongestants (such as the Vicks Inhaler). If sensitive detection techniques are used, use of nasal inhalers can produce a urine that is "positive" for methamphetamine.

Chapter 2
ENDNOTES

1. D. C. DesJarlais and S. R. Friedman, "Intravenous Cocaine, Crack, and HIV Infections," (letter) *Journal of the American Medical Association* 259 (1988): 1945-46.

2. R. L. Ritzgerald et al., "Resolution of Methamphetamine Stereoisomers in Urine Drug Testing: Urinary Excretion of R(-)Methamphetamine Following Use of Nasal Inhalers," *Journal of Analytical Toxicology* 12 (1988): 255-59.

3
MEDICAL COMPLICATIONS
OF METHAMPHETAMINE AND COCAINE USE

Smoking methamphetamine or freebase cocaine can cause many serious medical complications. There is an enormous amount of literature about the medical complications of cocaine and methamphetamine abuse. For this overview, we have selected key recent references that review medical complications or references to the first reports of the complications.

The toxicity of cocaine or methamphetamine can come not only from the drugs themselves, but also from the materials used to "cut" the drugs, the residuals of chemicals used in their manufacture, and, for cocaine, the residuals of herbicides. Herbicides, sprayed in attempts to destroy coca plants, have been recovered in samples of coca leaves and coca paste.[1]

To counsel drug abusers about the risks of their drug use and to make appropriate medical referrals, counselors need to know the medical complications that may be produced by the use of crack, cocaine freebase, and ice.

Addicts do not always recognize that medical complications are *caused* by smoking stimulants and may attribute causality to stress, trauma, or other drug use. They may also think the medical complications occur only with intravenous drug use.

Physicians who treat the complications of stimulant abuse without knowledge of their patients' drug use may misdiagnose the cause of the complications. Since the complications for cocaine and methamphetamine are similar, we will compare and contrast them.

NEUROLOGICAL COMPLICATIONS

Seizures

Grand mal seizures are the most common type of seizure produced by smoking crack or cocaine freebase. One survey of

39

adolescent cocaine abusers reported that 1 to 10 percent of those who had smoked crack reported seizures.[2] Cocaine-induced grand mal seizures are no different in appearance from those produced by epilepsy. People who suffer grand mal seizures lose consciousness, fall to the ground, and undergo violent muscle jerking, often biting their tongue and losing control of their bladder. The seizures generally stop within a few minutes but can recur after several minutes. During seizures, victims may burn or cut themselves after falling on the smoking equipment and striking their head on a sharp object. The seizures often occur within minutes of smoking but can occur several hours after smoking cocaine when the levels of the drug are decreasing. Medical experts speculate that the seizures, which occur several hours after smoking, are caused by high levels of cocaine metabolites such as benzoylecgonine.

Addicts who have pre-existing epilepsy or who drink heavily may increase their risk of seizures. Repeated seizures may alter the brain such that there is an increased risk of seizures. Some medications, including antidepressants used for treatment of cocaine craving, may also increase the risk of seizures.

Stroke

Strokes in cocaine and methamphetamine abusers are almost always caused by rupturing arteries in the brain. Case reports of strokes resulting from cocaine and methamphetamine use are well-documented in medical journals.[3] The size of the ruptured artery and its location will determine the extent of brain injury. After an artery in the brain ruptures, the brain tissue that artery supplies with oxygen dies. Afterward, the damaged portion of brain may form scar tissue. This tissue may produce abnormal electrical activity that results in a permanent seizure disorder. If a large portion of brain tissue dies, the affected region liquifies. Should the liquified portion of the brain become infected, a brain abscess is formed.

Strokes are the result of transient rises in blood pressure that occur during stimulant smoking. These increases in pressure can be substantial and can produce strokes in anyone. Some people are particularly vulnerable to stroke, especially those with a pre-existing abnormality on an artery known as an aneurysm. An aneurysm is a portion of an artery whose wall is thinner than the surrounding artery. This thinner section balloons out from the main vessel. Aneurysms often occur where two arteries join together. Since the ballooned-out portion of the artery is the weakest point on the artery, it is the most vulnerable to rupture. Unfortunately, most people who have aneurysms do not know that they have them until they rupture.

PULMONARY COMPLICATIONS

Bronchitis

The smoke from crack is hot and irritating to the lungs. Crack smokers often have bronchitis and describe coughing up "black stuff" from their lungs.

Crack Lung

Physicians at Wayne State University reported a case history of a forty-seven-year-old black woman who developed fever and pneumonia following crack use.[4] Her condition appeared to be an allergic reaction. The physicians called it "crack lung." Other investigators have reported functional abnormalities in the lungs of crack smokers; however, most of the subjects in the study also smoked tobacco and marijuana, so there was question about ascribing the dysfunction solely to crack smoking.[5]

Rupture of Lung

Physicians at the Emory University School of Medicine in Atlanta, Georgia, reported three cases of pneumomediastinum (air in non-lung tissue of the chest) caused by crack smoking.[6] The patients complained of chest or neck pain occurring one to six hours after smoking crack. As is common when crack smokers seek medical treatment, they did not initially reveal their histories of crack smoking to the attending physician.

CARDIOVASCULAR COMPLICATIONS

Heart Attacks

Cocaine can cause substantial increases in heart rate and blood pressure. The rapidly pumping heart at increased arterial pressure has increased oxygen needs. If the arteries that supply blood (the source of oxygen) to the heart muscle cannot supply sufficient blood, the heart muscle can die. In medical terms, this is known as myocardial infarction, or more commonly known as a heart attack. Myocardial infarction has occurred in people smoking cocaine who did not have pre-existing heart disease.

INFECTIONS

HIV Infection

Cocaine and methamphetamine are associated with HIV infection in two ways. First, shared-needle use is common among IV stimulant users and carries a major risk for transmission of HIV. Second, stimulant use for some is associated with high-risk sexual practices, because of both high-risk sexual behavior and the exchange of sex for drugs.

SEXUAL DYSFUNCTION

Cocaine and methamphetamine alter sexual functioning in both men and women. Men usually value the effects of cocaine on sexual functioning more than women. Many men value stimulants because they typically increase sexual desire. In men who are not chronic users, small doses typically increase sexual desire and delay ejaculation. However, the cocaine also makes getting an erection more difficult. In high doses or with chronic cocaine use, getting an erection may become impossible.

This increase in sexual desire is much less frequent in women who use cocaine and methamphetamine. With small amounts of stimulant, they may be less sexually inhibited but have difficulty with vaginal lubrication and with achieving orgasm. With higher doses, orgasm may become impossible.

For some methamphetamine abusers, sexual functioning and drug use are closely linked. People who use amphetamine at high doses report that their sexual desire and performance are enhanced.[7] This enhanced sexual desire is associated with increased sexual fantasy, leading to deviant sexual practices. This, in turn, can lead to high-risk sexual practices.[8] In males, the increase in sexual performance is characterized by delayed ejaculation. Gay males who often use amphetamines in high-risk sexual situations are at increased risk for HIV disease.

Continued abuse of methamphetamine, particularly when combined with alcohol, can produce sexual dysfunction, including erectile failure in males and desire-phase disorder in females. The enhancer becomes the inhibitor as the disease of addiction progresses. Someone in the early stage of recovery from addiction may have difficulty functioning sexually without amphetamine. A desire to enhance sexual function may be a significant relapse issue in early recovery.[9]

Decrease in Sperm Count

A study of 1,309 males conducted at the Yale University School of Medicine in New Haven, Connecticut, found that monthly or more frequent cocaine use was associated with a low sperm count. Those who had used cocaine five or more years had a higher frequency of low sperm counts, low sperm motility, and a larger number of abnormally formed sperm.[10] Subjects in the study were predominantly white males thirty-one to thirty-five years old.

PREGNANCY

Crack Babies

A distressing aspect of the crack epidemic is the large number of infants delivered to crack-dependent or crack-using mothers.

Kaye et al. report that birth outcomes for infants of crack abusers were worse than for infants of mothers who abused other forms of cocaine.[11] The outcomes were worse, especially in terms of lower birth weight and increased incidence of adverse neurological signs.

In reviewing the literature on cocaine abuse in pregnancy from 1982 to 1989, Lindenberg et al. presented a recap of the effects of cocaine abuse on obstetrical, neonatal, infant health, and development outcomes.[12] With regard to obstetrical outcomes, they found that cocaine or crack abusers (compared to nonusers) were less likely to have received prenatal care, had poorer nutritional status, and were more likely to have obstetrical complications. These complications included preterm labor and delivery, premature rupture of membranes, anemia, and sexually transmitted diseases. For newborns, outcomes included such complications as fetal distress in labor and delivery, low birth weight, neonatal withdrawal, congenital malformations, and sudden infant death. Adverse outcomes related to infant health and development included lower gestational age, birth weight, birth length, and head circumference in cocaine-exposed infants.

These "crack babies" often have severe neurological and developmental problems. Chasnoff and colleagues at the Northwestern University medical school in Chicago warned of the neurophysiological aftereffects (sequelae) of in utero cocaine exposure.[13] They also found a marked increase (15 percent) of Sudden Infant Death Syndrome (SIDS) in infants born to mothers who had used cocaine during pregnancy.

Subsequent publications have described other adverse effects of cocaine. Wang and Schnoll reported reductions in the placenta's receptor binding of some common neurotransmitters.[14] Recently, a letter in the publication *Pediatrics* raised the subject of the possibility of congenital malformations.[15]

The December 1991 issue of *Science* reported on the research findings of William Lyman at the Albert Einstein College of Medicine, linking cocaine use with vasculitis, "which may permit leaks between the fetal and maternal blood supply."[16]

Chasnoff, Griffith, and MacGregor compared perinatal outcomes of women who used cocaine throughout pregnancy with those of women who used cocaine only during the first trimester.[17] Infants exposed to cocaine throughout pregnancy had a low birth weight and an increased rate of preterm delivery and intrauterine growth retardation. Infants in both groups demonstrated significant neurobehavioral impairment.

Spence et al. found that "women with positive urines were almost four times as likely to have pre-term labor and over twice as likely to deliver a premature infant or one with a one-minute Apgar score of six or lower."[18]*

Sturner and colleagues reported six cases of cocaine-related infant deaths.[19] In each case, positive toxicological urine screens confirmed the presence of cocaine or metabolites in the mother's or baby's urine at birth. These infants, who came under the jurisdiction of the medical examiner, "had toxic exposure during maternal cocaine intoxication and have succumbed in utero, have been severely damaged at birth, or have been placed in other risk categories—including homicide—as developing babies."

Infants exposed to cocaine postnatally through their mothers' breast milk may exhibit numerous adverse effects, including irritability, high-pitched crying, tachycardia, hypertension, tremulousness, vomiting, diarrhea, dilated pupils, increased startles, and

---

*The Apgar score is an evaluation of a newborn infant's well-being and ability to survive, based on the infant's heart rate, breathing, muscle tone, reflexes, and color. Each factor is scored from a low value of 0 to a normal value of 2, and then those scores are combined. The higher the score, the healthier the baby, with 10 being the highest composite score. Typically, the assessments are done at one minute and five minutes after birth. The Apgar score is useful as a predictive measure of neonatal difficulties.

marked lability of mood.[20] Lewis also identifies the prenatal drug-exposed (PDE) toddler as being "at risk for a multitude of developmental concerns, including social, emotional, behavioral, and language problems [which] in turn place the PDE toddler at high risk for educational and social failure."

Pitts and Weinstein reviewed the adverse birth outcomes of perinatal cocaine exposure and concluded that "these children will require many years of observation to define developmental problems. Subtle learning disabilities and personality defects will become apparent only as the children grow older."[21]

Problems Beyond the Neonatal Period

Kelly, Walsh, and Thompson reported that in addition to having adverse birth outcomes, children of cocaine-using mothers were at greater risk for health problems beyond the neonatal period and also were at increased risk of being neglected and abused.[22] Cocaine infants have low thresholds for overstimulation, poor orientation to face and voice, and poor motor abilities. They attempt to shut out external stimulation. Their mothers may interpret this as personal rejection, reinforcing the mother's pre-existing low self-esteem, and it may foster ambivalent or hostile feelings on the part of the mother toward the infant. Given their health problems and limited interactive skills, these infants may be difficult to parent. Some cocaine-using mothers are known to neglect and mistreat their offspring. More cocaine-exposed children than those not exposed to cocaine were placed in foster homes because of maternal neglect.

Neglect and abuse of infants are common among crack-abusing mothers, and there is little that can be done to protect the infants. The numbers of infants affected has overwhelmed County Child Protective Services in many cities. Neighborhoods where crack is prevalent have become so hazardous for agency workers that they are refusing to make home visits.

Many of these crack-dependent mothers are Black, and since many Blacks are of lower socioeconomic status they would

46

ordinarily receive their medical treatment in county and other public hospitals. But treatment of crack-dependent mothers is not confined to the public sector. In California, at least, the most economically disadvantaged have access to private hospitals through Medi-Cal, California's Medicaid program, or county contracts. In some instances, the women arrive at the hospital emergency room in labor, and the hospital must provide care, regardless of the women's ability to pay.

In Oakland and surrounding East Bay cities, despite the large numbers of infants born to cocaine-dependent mothers, despite the high cost of providing intensive care and foster care placement for many of the infants, and despite rampant local concern about the crack epidemic among women, there is still little drug abuse treatment available to mothers who are crack-dependent.

Use of smokable methamphetamine can produce difficulties similar to crack. "Ice babies" are common in areas such as Hawaii, the Philippines, and Korea, where the smoking of ice is prevalent. If ice use becomes prevalent in the United States, we will also see increasing numbers of infants affected by that drug.

DEATH

The Drug Abuse Warning Network of the National Institute on Drug Abuse collects medical examiners' reports of drug-related deaths. In 1988, coroners across the United States attributed 2,254 deaths to cocaine. In 1989, there were 2,496 deaths attributed to cocaine.[23] Figure 3.1 on the next page compares cocaine- and heroin-related deaths reported to NIDA during 1988 and 1989.

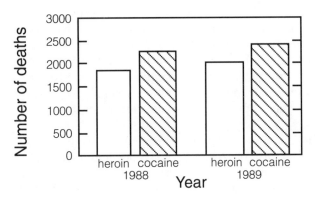

Fig. 3.1. Comparison of heroin- and cocaine-related deaths reported to NIDA's Drug Abuse Warning Network.

Chapter 3
ENDNOTES

1. M. A. Klosohly et al., "Analysis of 2, 4, - Dichlorophen- oxyacetic Acid in Coca Leaves and Coca Paste When the Herbicide Is Used to Control Coca Plants," *Bulletin Narcotics* 35 (1983): 67.
2. R. H. Schwartz, "Seizures Associated with Smoking 'Crack'— A Survey of Adolescent 'Crack' Smokers," (letter) *Western Journal of Medicine* 150 (1989): 213.
3. L. I. Golbe and M. D. Merkin, "Cerebral Infarction in a User of Free-Base Cocaine ('Crack')," *Neurology* 36 (1986): 1602-4. S. R. Levine et al., "Crack Cocaine Associated Stroke," *Neurology* 37 (1987): 1849-53.
4. D. G. Kissner et al., "Crack Lung: Pulmonary Disease Caused by Cocaine Abuse," *American Review of Respiratory Diseases* 136 (1987): 1250-52.
5. J. Itkonen, S. Schnoll, and J. Glassroth. "Pulmonary Dysfunction in 'Freebase' Cocaine Users," *Archives of Internal Medicine* 144 (1984): 2195-97.

6. S. L. Brody, G. V. Anderson Fr., and J. B. Gutman, "Pneumo-mediastinum as a Complication of 'Crack' Smoking," *American Journal of Emergency Medicine* 6 (1988): 241-43.

7. G. R. Gay et al., "Drug-Sex Practice in the Haight-Ashbury or 'the Sensuous Hippie'," in *Sexual Behavior—Pharmacology and Biochemistry*, ed. M. Sandler and G. Gessa (New York: Raven Press, 1975); F. H. Gawin, "Drugs and Eros: Reflections on Aphrodisiacs," *Journal of Psychedelic Drugs* 10 (1978).

8. D. E. Smith, M. E. Buxton, and G. Dammonn, "Amphetamine Abuse and Sexual Dysfunction: Clinical and Research Considerations," in *Amphetamine Use, Misuse, and Abuse: Proceedings of the National Conference*, 1978, ed. D. E. Smith, D. R. Wesson et al. (Boston: G. K. Hall, 1979): 228-48.

9. D. E. Smith, D. R. Wesson, and M. Apter-Marsh, "Cocaine- and Alcohol-Induced Sexual Dysfunction in Patients with Addictive Disease," *Journal of Psychoactive Drugs* 16 (1984): 359-61.

10. M. B. Bracken et al., "Association of Cocaine Use with Sperm Concentrations, Motility, and Morphology," *Fertility and Sterility* 53 (1990): 315.

11. K. Kaye et al., "Birth Outcomes for Infants of Drug Abusing Mothers," *New York State Journal of Medicine* 89 (1989): 256-61.

12. C. S. Lindenberg et al., "A Review of the Literature on Cocaine Abuse in Pregnancy," *Nursing Research* 40 (1991): 69-75.

13. I. J. Chasnoff, K. A. Burns, and W. J. Burns, "Cocaine Use in Pregnancy: Perinatal Morbidity and Mortality," *Neurotoxicology and Teratology* 9 (1987): 291-93.

14. C. H. Wang and S. H. Schnoll, "Prenatal Cocaine Use Associated with Down Regulation of Receptors in Human Placenta," *Neurotoxicology and Teratology* 9 (1987): 301-4.

15. J. Bays, "Fetal Vascular Disruption with Prenatal Exposure to Cocaine or Methamphetamine" (letter), *Pediatrics* 87 (1991): 416-17.

16. J. Palca, "HIV Risk Higher for First-Born Twins," *Science* 254 (1991): 1729.
17. I. J. Chasnoff et al., "Temporal Patterns of Cocaine Use in Pregnancy: Perinatal Outcome," *Journal of the American Medical Association* 261 (1989): 1741-44.
18. M. R. Spence et al., "The Relationship Between Recent Cocaine Use and Pregnancy Outcomes," *Obstetrics and Gynecology* 78 (1991): 326-29.
19. W. Q. Sturner et al., "Cocaine Babies: The Scourge of the '90s," *Journal of Forensic Sciences* 36 (1991): 34-39.
20. K. D. Lewis, "Pathophysiology of Prenatal Drug-Exposure: In Utero, in the Newborn, in Childhood, and in Agencies," *Journal of Pediatric Nursing* 6 (1991): 185-90.
21. K. S. Pitts and L. Weinstein, "Cocaine and Pregnancy—A Lethal Combination," *Journal of Perinatology* 10 (1990): 180-82.
22. S. J. Kelly, J. H. Walsh, and K. Thompson, "Birth Outcomes, Health Problems, and Neglect with Prenatal Exposure to Cocaine," *Periatric Nursing* 17 (1991): 130-36.
23. K. H. Sobel, "Cocaine-Related Hospital Emergency Room Visits Drop 30 Percent," *NIDA Notes* 5 (1990): 6-7. This is a national sample, but the national totals are actually higher because not all cocaine-related deaths are reported to NIDA.

4
PSYCHIATRIC COMPLICATIONS

Extensive literature reports a high prevalence of psychopathology among stimulant abusers. Psychopathology is an important issue for several reasons:

1. Underlying psychopathology may increase an individual's vulnerability to developing drug dependency.
2. Stimulant abusers with severe psychopathology, such as schizophrenia, have limited psychosocial treatment options and it is necessary to involve mental health professionals in their treatment.
3. High levels of psychopathology in drug abusers are generally associated with poor treatment outcome.
4. Psychopathology may predispose drug abusers to relapse.

Unraveling cause and effect in a stimulant abuser who begins drug use at an early age is not always possible, so treatment must be directed at both the psychopathology and the drug abuse disorder.

STIMULANT PSYCHOSES

Intoxication

People using large quantities of either cocaine or methamphetamine over a few hours can become so intoxicated that they rapidly become increasingly suspicious and develop delusional beliefs. In its extreme form, stimulant intoxication can produce a state that closely mimics paranoid schizophrenia.[1] While intoxicated, stimulant users may hear nonexisting voices or noises or misinterpret sounds as having special meaning. They may also develop false beliefs (such as that police cars are circling their house) and perceive that events relate to them that do not. For example, stimulant abusers may hear laughter outside a window and believe that the people outside are laughing at them (also called "ideas of reference").

During their intoxicated state, users may not recognize that their altered perception is drug-induced. Later, after the drug effect has stopped, users may remember some of their delusions and recognize them as having been drug-induced. The mental changes induced by stimulants have been studied experimentally and can occur even in people who have no underlying psychiatric disorder.[2]

Long-Lasting Effects of Stimulants

People who abuse stimulants over months or years and repeatedly become intoxicated can develop prolonged alterations in their brain functioning. These include:

1. exacerbation or intensification of symptoms in schizophrenics
2. precipitation of latent schizophrenia
3. prolonged psychosis following an episode of acute stimulant psychosis
4. sensitization to stimulant-induced psychosis

Stimulant-induced psychosis is often misdiagnosed as schizophrenia. Stimulant abusers who are paranoid often deny that they are using drugs. Unless their stimulant use is detected with a drug screen, the drug abuser will be diagnosed as a paranoid schizophrenic.

ANXIETY REACTIONS

Panic Attacks

Panic disorders are a subgroup of anxiety disorders. Panic attacks typically begin with the sudden onset of intense fear or terror. They may last minutes to hours. A real panic attack is not a phobic response triggered by environmental cues. A person having a panic attack may experience trembling, sweating, chest pain, abdominal pain, or difficulty breathing. Often the person feels that he or she is either going crazy or dying. Although someone who is intoxicated by a stimulant may experience severe anxiety, fear, or some of the same symptoms of a panic attack, he or she should not be diagnosed as suffering a panic attack while under the influence of drugs.

Case reports suggest that crack cocaine may produce a panic disorder.[3] It is important that the counselor be able to recognize a true panic disorder, because medication treatment (such as a tricyclic antidepressant like imipramine or a benzodiazepine) can sometimes stop the attacks.

Stimulant users may not know that their panic attacks are caused by their stimulant use, and they may self-medicate their attacks with street drugs or alcohol.

Chapter 4
ENDNOTES

1. D. S. Bell, "A Comparison of Amphetamine Psychosis and Schizophrenia," *British Journal of Psychiatry* 3 (1965): 701-6.
2. T. H. Connell, *Amphetamine Psychosis* (London: Chapman and Hall, 1958); B. M. Angrist and S. Gershon, "The Phenomenology of Experimentally Induced Amphetamine Psychosis: Preliminary Observations," *Biological Psychiatry* 2 (1970): 95-107; J. D. Griffith et al., "Dextroamphetamine: Evaluation of Psychomimetric Properties in Man," *Archives of General Psychiatry* 26 (1972): 97-100; E. H. Ellinwood, "Amphetamine Psychosis: Description of the Individuals and Process," *Journal of Nervous and Mental Disorders* 144 (1967): 273-83.
3. W. A. Price and A. J. Giannini, "Phencyclidine and 'Crack' Precipitated Panic Disorder" (letter), *American Journal of Psychiatry* 144 (1987): 686-87; H. D. Abraham, "Do Psychostimulants Kindle Panic Disorder?" *American Journal of Psychiatry* 133 (1986): 627-34; T. A. Aronson and T. J. Craig, "Cocaine Precipitation of Panic Disorder," *American*

Journal of Psychiatry 143 (1986): 1320; R. Pohl, R. Balon, and V. K. Yeragani, "More on Cocaine and Panic Disorder," *American Journal of Psychiatry* 144 (1987): 1363.

5
TREATMENT MODALITIES

A variety of modalities can be used for treatment of stimulant abuse. The importance of matching patients to the most appropriate modality cannot be overemphasized. Timing is also crucial, because the patient's needs often change as treatment progresses. In this chapter, we describe treatment modalities and give practical guidelines for deciding on the most useful modalities at specific points in a patient's recovery process.

Because most stimulant abusers will have significant medical, psychological, economic, relationship, and legal problems in addition to their drug problem, they may require simultaneous or sequential use of various types of modalities. At first, meeting the required needs can seem overwhelming, particularly since patients generally want all their needs met at once. For this reason, it is important to develop a written treatment plan as a guide for both the patient and the counselor.

DEVELOPING THE TREATMENT PLAN

The first step in developing a treatment plan is to assess the patient's problems comprehensively, determine what treatment modalities are acceptable to the patient, and define the resources that are accessible to the patient. The assessment may need to be carried out over several meetings with the patient.

The problem assessment should include:

- need for detoxification
- active medical illnesses
- difficulties at work
- pending criminal charges or legal proceedings
- pressing financial problems
- drug use in the family

- the patient's living environment
- psychological problems

Once problems have been identified, they need to be prioritized according to problems that must be dealt with immediately and those that can be addressed later. The problems needing immediate attention are those that must be resolved if the patient's drug use is to be interrupted.

The second step is to identify resources accessible to the patient. The operative word is "accessible." Accessibility is most often limited by economic considerations. For most patients treated in publicly funded programs, economic considerations severely restrict the patient's access to many types of treatment. At the Haight-Ashbury Free Clinics, for example, most patients coming to treatment do not have health insurance.

The final step is to negotiate with the patient a plan that is acceptable, given the resources that are accessible to the patient.

Detoxification

Stimulant abuse itself does not usually require detoxification medications; however, stimulant abusers often require detoxification from sedatives. Most stimulant abusers eventually become heavy users of some kind of depressant: alcohol, marijuana, benzodiazepines (Valium or Valium-like sedatives), or opiates, such as heroin. The phenomenon is not unique to users of smokable stimulants, but is an almost predictable consequence of long-term, high-dose stimulant abuse, regardless of the mode of use. During the epidemic of injectable methamphetamine abuse in the Haight-Ashbury from 1969 to 1972, we often observed methamphetamine abusers who developed a secondary dependency on opiates or heroin.[1] In the mid-to-late 1970s, when cocaine freebase use became fashionable among the wealthy in Marin County (an upper-class suburb north of San Francisco), many people began mixing freebase with Persian heroin and developed a primary heroin dependency. They were often surprised when they developed heroin withdrawal symptoms, because they erroneously believed they could not become dependent on heroin unless they injected it.

If the patient has a secondary dependency on opiates, alcohol, or benzodiazepines, he or she must be detoxified before beginning primary treatment of the stimulant abuse. Untreated, or improperly treated, sedative-hypnotic withdrawal can be life-threatening. Withdrawal protocols for treatment of sedative-hypnotic and alcohol dependency are beyond the scope of this book. We and others have previously published protocols for withdrawal of sedative-hypnotics[2] and opiates.[3]

Resolving Medical Problems

Many stimulant abusers have serious medical problems that must be addressed early in treatment. Unless they have access to mainstream medical treatment, their medical problems often must be managed in the drug treatment clinic. In effect, drug treatment clinics have become health maintenance organizations (HMOs) for addicts on the lower end of the socioeconomic scale. A recognition that drug treatment clinics provide primary medical care for many patients with infectious diseases (such as TB, hepatitis, and AIDS) has been a driving force for federal funding of drug treatment clinics.

Treatment of Stimulant Abuse in Public Sector Programs

Once the acute medical and psychiatric problems have been stabilized and the patient has been detoxified from secondary sedative-hypnotics or opiates, the focus of treatment can shift to primary treatment of stimulant abuse. In public sector programs, such as the Haight-Ashbury Free Clinic, most patients enter a recovery group.[4] While there are many variants of the recovery group, they all have relapse prevention as a major goal and incorporate concepts of relapse prevention developed in treatment of alcoholism.[5]

Recovery-Sensitive Counseling

Patients often need individual counseling to address issues not easily discussed in the group. There are two reasons why groups cannot handle all issues. First, a patient may be uncomfortable discussing certain issues if he or she is the only member of the group with the particular problem. Second, depending on the makeup of the group, some topics may generate controversy and discomfort among the members. The group consensus soon labels them taboo topics—topics best addressed in individual counseling sessions. For example, patients whose stimulant abuse was part of their sexual practice may need specific sexual counseling.

The Role of Twelve Step Recovery

Twelve Step recovery work often complements work within the recovery group. Whether a particular patient will do best in Alcoholics Anonymous or Cocaine Anonymous depends more on the makeup of the group and a patient's lifestyle than on what the particular group is called. Patients who are not antagonistic toward religion and whose lifestyle is mainstream often are more comfortable in Alcoholics Anonymous. The important point is that members of recovery groups attend different Twelve Step meetings and discover what is most helpful for them.

THERAPEUTIC COMMUNITIES

In substance abuse treatment, therapeutic communities were developed primarily as a way of treating heroin dependency. Therapeutic communities should be a major form of treatment for many crack-dependent people. Many of these communities are currently adapting their services for stimulant abusers, and some of these adaptations include a greater acceptance of mental health services and psychotherapeutic medications.

Many crack users come from homes where their spouse or other family members are still using crack. It is unrealistic to expect most of the recovering people to remain abstinent for any significant time if they return to that kind of an environment. For such individuals, six months to a year in a therapeutic community offers the best chance of reaching a stable abstinence.

PSYCHOTHERAPY

The role of psychotherapy, in any of its forms, in treatment of drug abuse continues to spark controversy. Psychotherapy alone is unlikely to be sufficient treatment for someone still abusing drugs. On the other hand, psychotherapy can be useful in conjunction with drug abuse treatment. We will describe the more noteworthy features of some common psychotherapies and give guidelines for their use in the treatment of stimulant abusers.

Empirical evidence for the effectiveness of psychotherapy in treatment of drug abuse is difficult to obtain. Research in psychotherapeutic effectiveness is extremely difficult because (1) the patient and therapist always know which treatment is being given, and (2) the personality and skill of the therapist can affect treatment retention and outcome.

Analytic Psychotherapy

Freudian psychoanalysis differs from other psychotherapeutic approaches in that analysis of the patient's transference to the analyst is the central task. Therapeutic benefit is assumed to derive from insight into reactions the patient has to the therapist. The therapy is structured to encourage the patient's development of transference. The therapist provides little personal information, and in formal psychoanalysis the patient lies on a couch and the therapist sits behind the patient. The frequency of sessions ranges from one to five times a week.

Psychoanalysis usually causes anxiety in the patient, which is not helpful to someone who has abused drugs to avoid anxiety or conflict. Patients sometimes use drugs before the analytic session or immediately afterward to reduce the anxiety induced by the session.

The anxiety can be a problem for patients in early abstinence, and analytic psychotherapy itself can result in relapse if more anxiety is induced than the patient can tolerate. In our experience, analysts often overestimate the capacity of their patients in early abstinence to deal with discomfort. For this reason, we generally advise against psychoanalytic work during early recovery. Later, however, analysis can benefit some patients. Our guidelines are as follows:

- Patients are advised not to initiate psychoanalytic therapy until they have had at least a year of comfortable abstinence from all abuse of drugs, including alcohol.
- Patients with the following characteristics are good analytic candidates:
    1. They began their drug abuse in their late twenties or into their thirties.
    2. They have had considerable educational and work accomplishments.
    3. They successfully make and keep friends.
    4. They are verbal and curious about why they feel what they feel.

BEHAVIOR THERAPY

One common theory of relapse holds that drug abusers relapse in response to drug cravings induced by certain objects, people, or situations. By repeatedly experiencing drug-induced euphoria paired with certain objects, people, or situations, the stimulant abuser becomes conditioned to associate the objects, people, or situations with stimulant use. When these factors are subsequently encountered, cravings for stimulants are "triggered." This form of "learning" is often referred to as "classical" or "Pavlovian" conditioning.

Classical conditioning is the basis of most advertising and can occur without conscious awareness. An ad designer may repeatedly pair a product with something potential consumers already find desirable, so consumers "learn" that the product is also desirable.

Therapeutic modalities designed to directly alter conditioned learning are often called "behavior" therapies. Behavior therapies can be *aversive conditioning*, in which the drug or drug-use equipment is paired repeatedly with nausea or electric shock; or *deconditioning*, in which the drug or drug-use equipment is paired with relaxation. Although both treatments have as their ultimate goals the reduction of drug use, the intermediate goals are different. With aversive conditioning, the goal is to produce an active aversion in the patient to the drug or drug-use situation. With deconditioning, the goal is to extinguish the patient's conditioned responses to the drug or drug-use situation.

The most well-known aversive behavior therapy for drug abuse is emetine, used for treatment of alcoholism. Ingestion of emetine produces nausea. In treatment, detoxified alcohol abusers are first made to feel nauseated by taking emetine, then allowed to smell and taste their favorite alcoholic beverage. Repeated pairing of nausea with the smell and taste of alcohol produces an aversion to alcohol. Emetine therapy has also been used with cocaine. The patient is allowed to handle cocaine-use paraphernalia while nauseated.

Other behavior therapies used for cocaine dependence are also classified as "deconditioning." The purpose is to reverse the conditioning that has built up during the time the person was using cocaine. With repeated use of cocaine, the user develops "conditioned" physiological responses (such as increased heart rate) to the sight, smell, or thought of cocaine. Conditioning also occurs when the user associates (or pairs) being high with the paraphernalia used to get high. These physiological responses may contribute to craving. To decondition the response, the cocaine abuser is repeatedly shown pictures of, and is allowed to handle, cocaine pipes or other equipment while in a state of deep relaxation. With time, the patient's conditioned physiological responses are extinguished.

Studies demonstrate that addicts can decondition their physiological response by handling drug use equipment and seeing videos of other people using drugs. The efficacy of deconditioning therapy in producing long-term decreases in cocaine use, however, has not been satisfactorily established.

ACUPUNCTURE

Acupuncture as a treatment for crack dependency has stimulated much interest. Electrical acupuncture is a low-cost treatment option because it can be administered to many patients concurrently by one technician.[6]

SPECIALIZED TREATMENT SERVICES FOR MOTHERS

There are few services available for addicted or drug-using pregnant women. Because of liability concerns, most drug treatment programs actively discourage pregnant women from getting treatment. Unless prenatal services are provided at the treatment clinic, many stimulant-abusing women who are pregnant receive no prenatal care. They actively avoid medical care for fear that their stimulant abuse will be discovered and their infant will be taken from them. The women, however, are at extreme risk for developing complications during their pregnancy. Lack of prenatal care, poor diet, the vasoconstrictor effect of high-dose cocaine and amphetamine on the placenta, and the lifestyle of the drug abusers combine to put the infant at high risk for complications. However, there have been noteworthy attempts to provide specialized treatment services for pregnant women who are addicted.

Therapeutic Communities for Women

Mandela House, a five-bed residential program in East Oakland, California, is one approach to providing services to pregnant, crack-using women. It was started by a Black woman, Minnie Thomas, and was the subject of an article in *Time* magazine.[7] Residential programs like Mandela House are important because they provide a drug-free environment. Treatment for some addicts becomes irrelevant if they have to return to an environment where they will be tempted to use again. Places such as these offer a protected environment for both the mother and the infant. They also provide a place for a woman to learn basic parenting skills and basic life skills for managing and coping once she leaves the protected environment. Places such as Mandela House are few and far between, and waiting lists are long.

The Haight-Ashbury Free Clinics have a somewhat similar program called Smith House for homeless alcohol-addicted women. Smith House works with the Clinics' Women's Needs Center and MAMA (Moving Addicted Mothers Ahead) Project, providing specialized services for female addicts and their children.

Specialized recovery houses such as these also provide a therapeutic environment away from the drug culture. A woman's motivation for treatment often emanates from her desire to reconnect with her children and to escape a chemically dependent, abusive relationship. A specialized recovery center for women provides them with a healthy alternative to a destructive lifestyle while they deal with the specific issues needed to begin a recovery program.

MEDICATION TREATMENT

The difficulty of keeping crack users in outpatient programs and the high relapse rate of crack users following inpatient programs have driven clinicians to search for medications that might improve treatment outcome. Until recently, most of the investigation into medications for treatment of drug abuse was conducted by individual researchers, sometimes with grant support from NIDA. This is unusual because most medication development for treatment of illnesses in the United States is conducted by pharmaceutical companies. The reason medications for treatment of drug abuse have been developed outside pharmaceutical companies is that most companies are reluctant to have their medications even remotely associated with the treatment of substance abuse.

Pharmaceutical companies have shunned the drug abuse field for several reasons. First, developing medication is enormously expensive and time-consuming. The Pharmaceutical Manufacturer's Association estimates that the average medication takes ten years and $125 million in research and development costs before it is available for physicians to prescribe. To make the medication development process profitable for a pharmaceutical company, the medication must have a large potential market. In pharmaceutical market terms, the total number of drug abusers is small. Therefore, companies are unwilling to commit their resources to developing treatments for drug abusers. Furthermore, there is the difficulty of doing reliable research with drug abusers. They don't comply in following a study protocol, and the accuracy of the information they give to researchers is questionable.

Second, pharmaceutical companies do not want their current products to be used for treatment of drug abusers. Because drug abusers are at high risk for misusing medication, they are at high risk for medical complications, which could result in product liability suits against the drug companies. In addition, physicians may be reluctant to prescribe a medication associated with drug abusers. This is because media publicity about its use in treatment for chemical dependency may cause other patients to be reluctant to take the medication.

While the problem with pharmaceutical companies is still a major issue, there has been some success. The Orphan Drug Act of 1983 provides tax incentives for companies that develop medications for a limited market. The act also gives the companies a seven-year exclusive on the medications during which no other company can market that product.[8] While this has helped in developing medication for the treatment of some rare medical conditions, it has not yet resulted in new medications for treatment of drug abuse.

Most research of medications for treating drug abuse is conducted by physicians working alone or in small groups. Often, these physicians apply for a grant from NIDA to support their research. This physician-initiated medication development has advantages and disadvantages. The main advantages of these researchers are the quickness and flexibility they have in responding to specific patient needs.

The disadvantages, however, are many and continue to plague the substance abuse treatment field, particularly when it comes to treatment of stimulant abusers. Development studies usually involve a relatively small number of subjects, and the statistical analysis and presentation of data are not always rigorous. The interest in new treatments for drug abuse is high, both within the drug abuse treatment community and among the general scientific and lay press. Because of this high interest, these studies often receive media exposure far beyond their importance. A disadvantage may be that clinicians prescribe medications whose safety and efficacy are not clearly established.

In the future, medication development for treatment of drug abuse may break from the past. Congress has appropriated considerable funds for finding new medication treatments for substance abusers, and medication development has become a separate division at NIDA. By acting as a sponsor, the Medication Development Division of NIDA is assuming many of the functions of a pharmaceutical company in the usual drug development process.

MEDICATIONS FOR
TREATMENT OF COCAINE DEPENDENCE

Both NIDA's Medication Development Division and Treatment Research Division are conducting research on many medications for treatment of cocaine dependence. If the addition of medication to psychosocial treatments increases the numbers of cocaine abusers who are treated, improved retention of patients in treatment, or decreased the rate of relapse, medications will have an important adjunctive role in treatment of stimulant abuse.

Medications may be useful for the following purposes:

- to manage acute medical toxicity (e.g., high blood pressure, grand mal seizure) or psychiatric toxicity (e.g., paranoid psychosis)
- to reduce cocaine withdrawal symptoms
- to facilitate abstinence
- to reduce relapse

The use of medications in managing acute medical and psychiatric toxicity is well established. Emergency treatment or acute psychiatric intervention generally occurs in a medical or psychiatric hospital.

The primary difficulty is that these occasions are not always used to best advantage to get the patient to treatment for his or her cocaine abuse. Many patients clearly do not want, or are not ready for, drug abuse treatment, but a patient's denial is often shattered during the emergency episode. To miss this window of opportunity to intervene and engage the patient in treatment for cocaine dependence is tragic.

REDUCTION OF WITHDRAWAL SYMPTOMS

After an episode of heavy cocaine use, most people experience an acute withdrawal phase lasting one to five days. Common symptoms include anxiety, insomnia, irritability, exhaustion, and sadness. The withdrawal syndrome, obvious to users of cocaine long before a withdrawal syndrome was accepted by the medical profession, was commonly called the "cocaine blues" or a "crash." The unpleasant mood following heavy use of stimulants can have two components:

1. a physiological component produced by the exhaustion of neuro-transmitters (e.g., norepinephrine, dopamine, and serotonin)
2. a psychological component due to remorse over what the person did while intoxicated (e.g., money spent)

Patients must be carefully assessed for suicidal ideation during the several days following a cocaine binge, since many cocaine abusers have committed suicide during the "crash."

Medication treatment of the symptoms may make patients more comfortable and, in some instances, more accepting, of treatment. From a medical standpoint, medication treatment is not necessary, and no medication has established efficacy in treatment of cocaine withdrawal.

Facilitation of Abstinence

For economic reasons, most cocaine abusers are treated as out-patients. With outpatient treatment, treatment retention of stimulant abusers is generally poor, and relapse to cocaine use is common. A medication that would assist outpatients to stop using cocaine while in treatment would be of great practical importance. Desipramine and other antidepressants have been promoted and are used by clinicians for this purpose, but their usefulness is based on clinical impression rather than efficacy demonstrated in controlled clinical trials.

Relapse Prevention

Most patients can achieve abstinence from stimulants while hospitalized or sequestered in an environment in which stimulants are not readily available. Preventing relapse to stimulant use after weeks or months of abstinence is a different problem from "facilitating abstinence" among patients who have not achieved a significant period of abstinence. Physiological withdrawal symptoms and residual toxicity are less problematic after a period of abstinence.

The rationale for medication treatments is primarily driven by two models of relapse:

- Self-medication hypothesis: Relapse is thought to occur because patients are unable to tolerate symptoms of dysphoria and anxiety, or because they have lost the ability to experience normal pleasure (sometimes called "anhedonia"), and they use the drug to alleviate the symptoms.
- Cocaine craving hypothesis: Relapse is thought to occur when patients experience overwhelming cravings for cocaine. The cravings may be produced by cocaine-induced changes in brain chemistry *or* may be environmentally or situationally induced.

The two hypotheses need not be mutually exclusive. In the same person, relapse may be driven by self-medication of symptoms at one time and by conditioned cravings at another time.

CORRECTION OF UNDERLYING PSYCHOPATHOLOGY

One prominent psychiatric theory of relapse holds that relapse is driven by patients' underlying psychopathology, such as depression.

Drug abusers discover that stimulants temporarily relieve disturbing symptoms and that they "self-medicate" with stimulants when symptoms occur. Medication treatment in this model is directed to correct the underlying psychopathology. The theory is the basis of much antidepressant use for stimulant abusers.

Stimulant Antagonist

A medication that could block the euphoric effects of stimulants could be used to prevent relapse in the same way that naltrexone, which blocks the mood effects of heroin, is useful in preventing relapse to opiate use. A medication that would block the effects of cocaine or amphetamine remains a tantalizing theoretical possibility, but as yet, no potent cocaine blockers have been discovered.

Stimulant Substitute

An alternative to a stimulant blocker would be stimulant maintenance, analogous to methadone treatment for heroin dependence. The viability of maintenance as a practical treatment strategy for stimulant abuse is unknown. The small amount of available research has used methylphenidate, and the results are not encouraging.

Antidepressants

Many antidepressant medications have been used for treatment of cocaine dependence, and antidepressants are commonly prescribed for cocaine abusers by addiction medicine specialists. They have been used to facilitate abstinence, prevent relapse, reduce craving, and treat underlying depression.

Desipramine
Of the antidepressants, desipramine is the most widely prescribed and has received the most study.[9] Despite its widespread use and attention in the media, desipramine has not been scientifi-

cally established as effective for treatment of cocaine dependency. It may be helpful in treating cocaine abusers who have depression that is not caused by their cocaine abuse.

Amantadine

Use of cocaine depletes the brain of neurotransmitters such as dopamine, norepinephrine, and serotonin. Amantadine, used in treatment of Parkinsonism, facilitates the release of dopamine and delays the re-uptake of dopamine into the synaptic vesicles. It has been used to treat cocaine cravings[10] and to reduce cocaine craving in methadone-maintained patients who have abused cocaine.[11]

The side effects of amantadine include difficulty in thinking, confusion, light-headedness, and anxiety. It can cause cardiac problems and is unsafe for pregnant women or nursing mothers.

The use of amantadine for treatment of cocaine dependence has not been established by adequate clinical studies.

Bromocriptine

Bromocriptine stimulates the same receptor site as dopamine. Since cocaine depletes the brain of dopamine, treatment with bromocriptine should alleviate cravings if they are caused by the dopamine depletion. Dackis and Gold reported that bromocriptine (.625 mg) produced a prompt decrease in cocaine craving, whereas medications that antagonize dopamine increased cocaine craving.[12]

Bromocriptine has also been suggested for treatment of cocaine abusers with adult attention deficit disorders that preceded their use of cocaine.[13]

Although bromocriptine is potentially a useful adjunct, insufficient clinical studies exist at this time to establish the efficacy of it in treatment of cocaine dependence.

Buprenorphine

Buprenorphine, an opiate medication undergoing study as an alternative to methadone in treatment of opiate dependence, has been reported to suppress cocaine self-administration in rhesus monkeys.[14] One study in addicts suggests that buprenorphine might reduce cocaine use.[15] Data at this time are insufficient to establish the efficacy of buprenorphine as a treatment for cocaine dependence.

Methylphenidate

Methylphenidate is a stimulant medication used primarily to treat hyperactive children. Drawing on the model of methadone maintenance of opiate dependence, some investigators have considered whether controlled maintenance with a prescription stimulant would be practical for treatment of cocaine dependence. An initial case report suggested possible clinical usefulness.[16] Subsequent investigations have found, however, that methylphenidate may induce craving for cocaine. Methylphenidate should not be used with a cocaine abuser unless the patient has an attention deficit disorder that was present before cocaine abuse.[17]

Carbamazepine

Carbamazepine (Tegretol), an anticonvulsant used for treatment of epilepsy, has been reported to decrease cocaine craving in cocaine-abusing patients.[18]

Other Pharmacotherapies

Other medications, not available for prescription in the United States, are being investigated as possible treatment for cocaine abuse. Flupentixol decanoate is unique among these medications in that it is given by injection and its effects last over one week. A clinical study done in the Bahamas suggests that flupentixol may be effective in reducing cocaine craving.[19]

Current Status of Pharmacological Treatment

Although medication (particularly to reduce cocaine cravings) is commonly used in outpatient treatment programs, the efficacy of such treatment is not established. Since the neurochemical dysfunction associated with stimulant abuse will eventually dissipate without medication, it should be reserved for patients who are unable to remain abstinent without it.

For some patients, taking medication appears to help them remain abstinent and to participate in their recovery work. For others, it shifts the focus from doing their recovery work to "seeing if the medication works." To the extent that patients attribute their abstinence to the medication, they may be psychologically vulnerable to relapse when the medication is stopped.

INPATIENT AND OUTPATIENT TREATMENT

Inpatient versus outpatient treatment of cocaine dependency is an issue fraught with controversy. Although the arguments against inpatient care are couched in terms of the relative effectiveness of the two forms of treatment, it is important to understand that the real issue is reducing health care costs. At stake is the survival of hospital-based chemical dependency treatment. More importantly, with the focus on cost containment, the controversy misses the clinically relevant issue: which patients need hospital treatment?

In part, the situation was created by the drug abuse treatment providers. During the 1970s and early 1980s, hospital-based chemical dependency programs hospitalized for twenty-eight days or more all patients requiring treatment for their dependency. Inpatient treatment was the "cash cow" of most drug treatment services. If outpatient services were offered at all, they were subsidized by inpatient revenues.

We must also view the situation in the context of a much broader effort to contain *all* health care costs. Although chemical dependency treatment and mental health services are usually the first to be restricted, inpatient services for chemical dependency treatment have not been singled out. Inpatient services are also being restricted for many kinds of medical treatment, including renal dialysis and certain types of minor surgery.

The development is not all bad. In the past, many patients who were treated as inpatients may have been better served by less expensive, longer-term outpatient treatment. Many chemical dependency treatment programs now have both inpatient and outpatient treatment services, and staff must make a clinical decision about which patients should be hospitalized and which should be treated as outpatients.

Assigning patients to inpatient or outpatient treatment on the basis of the patient's need effectively dispenses with the controversy about the relative effectiveness of inpatient and outpatient treatment.

Erosion of the Disease Model

In addition, the disease model, which originated with alcoholism and was subsequently applied to other chemical dependencies, is losing support. The Supreme Court has ruled (Traynor vs. Turnage) that primary alcoholism constitutes "willful misconduct" with regard to particular Veterans Administration benefits. This decision reflects the growing trend to abandon the disease model of alcoholism in favor of a moral judgment model. While the Supreme Court claims it is not making a decision whether or not alcoholism is a disease (pointing out that authorities remain sharply divided on the issue), the Court's ruling, nonetheless, undermines the disease model.

The continued erosion of the disease model of alcoholism and, by association, other forms of drug dependency, has affected the way alcoholism and drug abuse are perceived by mainstream culture. Even more important, it has affected the willingness of insurance carriers to pay for treatment; that is, if chemical dependency is not a disease, then treatment is not a covered medical expense.

The cocaine abuse epidemic coincides with increasing efforts to contain cost in all areas of medicine, including addiction treatment services. Thus inpatient chemical dependency treatment, because of its conspicuous contribution to rising medical treatment costs, is being increasingly scrutinized by both the public and the private sectors. The dominant form of scrutiny comes from managed health care systems. During the past few years, managed health care has emerged as a method for containing costs and improving the allocation of health care resources. The providers of managed health care are positioned between the treatment service provider, the patient, and the insurance carrier. The health management group determines what services are needed, who can provide them, and who gets paid for providing them. Not surprisingly, case managers with managed health care groups view outpatient services as a less expensive alternative to inpatient treatment. For both the patient and the treatment provider, managed health care groups remove the opportunity to choose between treatment options. Instead, managed health care determines which option the patient must use and predominantly assigns outpatient treatment.

The Effectiveness Of
Inpatient vs. Outpatient Treatment

No controlled studies have been published comparing the effectiveness of inpatient vs. outpatient treatment of cocaine abusers; however, several such studies have been conducted in the treatment of alcoholism. In 1986, Miller and Hester published a meta-analysis of eight controlled studies comparing inpatient vs. outpatient treatment of alcoholism. From these studies, they concluded that inpatient programs do not result in any better outcome for the alcoholic population as a whole than does treatment on an outpatient basis.[20] A subsequent editorial in *Science* brought widespread attention to the Miller and Hester article.[21] Consequently, managed health care and insurance carriers often cite Miller and Hester's work to support restricted coverage of inpatient chemical dependency treatment.

Although the Miller and Hester studies use a control-group design, randomly assigning patients either to inpatient or outpatient treatment, studies are severely limited for a number of reasons. First is the inferred cause and effect relationship between a particular treatment episode and treatment outcome. Often patients have had more than one treatment episode for drug dependency. In the studies cited by Miller and Hester, however, it is assumed the outcome is determined only by the treatment episode being studied.

But many patients have multiple episodes of inpatient treatment, outpatient treatment, or both during their addiction career. The cumulative effect of multiple treatment episodes is unknown.

Further, clinicians commonly observe that patients fail to have more than a brief period of abstinence from drug use until some life circumstance profoundly changes their perception of their drug use and lifestyle. The circumstances that change people can vary enormously. For some, it may be finding themselves in the hospital for the fifth time, while for others it is a drug-induced illness, loss of a job, loss of a spouse, or death of a friend.

Whatever the cause, patients can vividly describe their turning point. Experienced clinicians and drug abuse counselors have a range of terms to describe the turning point. Those from the tradition of Alcoholics Anonymous call it "hitting bottom" or "breakdown of denial"; mental health professionals call it "insight."

There are also problems with the Miller and Hester studies that limit their ability to make generalizations about the treatment outcomes. Patients are not blind to the type of treatment they are receiving and may have strong feelings about whether they're getting the treatment they want, need, or deserve. Many subjects who are eligible for random assignment will either refuse treatment or drop out if assigned to a treatment they did not choose. Therefore, the studies' results are quite limited. The comparison of treatment outcome is, in fact, made on a *subset* of alcoholics that may be atypical in many ways: subjects who didn't need hospitalization for medical or psychiatric reasons, subjects who found their treatment assignment acceptable, subjects who completed treatment, and subjects who were available for follow-up. Thus to apply the findings to *all* alcoholics seeking treatment, let alone those who are addicted to other substances, is inappropriate.

The results of these studies are widely misused. Policymakers and insurance carriers justify excluding inpatient coverage because the studies did not find inpatient services more effective than outpatient. This type of thinking misses the point that inpatient and outpatient treatment are not competitive, but complementary. To ask which is more effective is like asking which tool contributes the most to building a house, a hammer or a saw? It's a ridiculous question. Hammers and saws are different tools, with different purposes, and both are needed to construct a house.

Treatment in the Past

All this controversy is positive because it forces treatment providers to reexamine their pattern of service delivery. In the past, most private providers hospitalized all chemically dependent patients in an inpatient treatment program. Following twenty-one to twenty-eight days in the inpatient program, the patient was discharged to aftercare, which typically included one or more group meetings a week for six months to two years and attendance at Cocaine Anonymous or some other Twelve Step recovery program.

Intensive inpatient treatment followed by a much less intense aftercare program is modeled after acute medical treatment. In the acute medical model, a patient is hospitalized during the illness and kept in the hospital until the needs for intravenous antibiotics and other specialized hospital services are no longer needed. The patient is then discharged and given a follow-up outpatient appointment. This will assure the patient and the physician that recovery is continuing on schedule. This model works well in acute, time-limited illnesses such as pneumonia.

When applied to drug dependence, however, the model has shortcomings. The model implies that the main part of treatment occurred during the inpatient stay and that aftercare is optional. In fact, the inpatient stay is crisis stabilization and treatment entry. The majority of the recovery work will come after the patient is discharged from the hospital. Recovery from serious drug dependency is a long-term process that takes years.

Inpatient Treatment

There are basically three types of hospitals that treat drug abusers:
- medical
- psychiatric
- chemical dependency recovery hospitals

An inpatient drug treatment program may, of course, be part of a medical or psychiatric hospital. But most often, inpatient chemical dependency treatment programs are in a separate building or ward. These programs also have a different staffing pattern than medical or psychiatric services. In California, chemical dependency recovery hospitals are a separate class of acute-care hospitals and have their own regulations regarding staffing and service delivery.

All three types of hospitals may have a role in treatment of stimulant abusers. Some patients may, in fact, require treatment in all three at different times.

To understand some of the current problems of treating stimulant abusers on an inpatient basis, it is helpful to have a broad, historical view of the modern hospital and to understand the social context in which hospitals operate.

A hospital is a highly specialized, highly regulated environment that brings together medical equipment, physicians, nurses, medical technicians, and other people with specialized expertise. This has not always been the case. Until the turn of this century, most hospitals were owned and operated by religious groups. There was little specialized equipment available, and the treatments available often did more harm than good. Patients were treated in hospitals not because they needed access to equipment or specialists, but rather because it was easier and more cost-effective to care for sick people together on a ward than to treat them at home. Inpatients were usually indigent and had no other access to medical care. Patients who could afford private care were usually not treated at a hospital, but at home.

The situation changed in great part because of advancing surgical and medical technology. Hospitals became places where specialized technology such as operating rooms, monitoring and diagnostic equipment, and increased levels of professional expertise could be concentrated and made available to patients.

All of this was accomplished at a high price. Inpatient treatment is astronomically expensive. The high costs result from the need for high-tech equipment, the specialized labor-intensive nature of the work, the need to meet the requirements of many state and federal regulatory agencies, and the awkwardness of insurance and other reimbursement mechanisms.

When chemical dependency treatment became hospital-based, chemical dependency programs inherited many of the costs associated with the modern hospital. With treatment of severe alcohol dependence, the costs could be justified in terms of medical need. But with treatment of stimulant abuse, which does not have a life-threatening withdrawal syndrome, the medical need is often not apparent.

Medical Hospitals

Many of the acute medical complications of stimulant abuse (e.g., stroke, myocardial infarction) require treatment in an inpatient medical hospital because of the serious, immediately life-threatening nature of the illness. The immediate medical or surgical care is no different for the stimulant abuser than for other patients. But once the acute, life-threatening aspects of the illness have been resolved, the physician and staff should expend every effort to motivate the patient for primary treatment of his or her stimulant or other drug abuse.

The following are guidelines for referral to a medical hospital:

- Treatment of patients' medical complications that cannot be treated on an outpatient basis because of the severity of the complication *or* because the erratic lifestyle of the patients makes it likely they will not follow through.
- Patients must be capable of cooperating with their treatment and be in control of their behavior so that they will not disrupt the care of other patients.

Psychiatric Hospitals

Psychiatric hospitals are useful because they can protect patients who are acutely suicidal or who are so delusional that they are likely to harm themselves or others. During acute stimulant psychosis, some patients are so delusional, impulsive, and behaviorally out of control that they must be treated for their medical condition in a psychiatric hospital. The level of behavioral control that can be imposed in a psychiatric hospital is virtually impossible in any other setting.

The following are guidelines for referral to a psychiatric hospital:

- Patients who are acutely suicidal.
- Patients who are homicidal because of stimulant-induced psychosis.
- Patients with medical complications and who are acutely psychotic and behaviorally unmanageable in an acute medical setting.
- Patients who, because of their stimulant abuse, are so disorganized they cannot arrange for their immediate food and shelter.

Chemical Dependency Recovery Hospitals

Most recovery-oriented chemical dependency inpatient treatment and some detoxification occur in specialized inpatient treatment units. In most states, these units are located within a medical or psychiatric hospital.

In California, chemical dependency treatment services are separately licensed. The treatment unit may be within an acute-care medical or psychiatric hospital, or it may be a free-standing hospital. The latter is called a chemical dependency recovery hospital (CDRH).

The staffing pattern of a CDRH differs from either a medical or psychiatric hospital. Many of the services are provided by substance abuse counselors, and there are fewer medical staff.

The following is a guideline for referral to a CDRH:

- Patients who are in need of the protected environment to remain drug-free and engage in recovery treatment services.

Short-Term Hospitalization

Most inpatient drug treatment programs have a specified length of stay, usually twenty-one or twenty-eight days. Knowing the length of stay before the patient is admitted has practical advantages for the patient and service provider but makes little sense clinically.

In a medical inpatient setting, the criteria for discharge are related to the disease process. Thus a patient with pneumonia is treated on an inpatient basis until the patient's signs and symptoms have improved. In treatment of psychiatric disorders, a patient who is admitted because of suicidal ideation may be discharged when the suicidal ideation, or the impulse to act on it, is no longer present.

Although the situation is somewhat different for cocaine-dependent patients, the principle remains the same. Discharge should be determined by patients' progress, not by the time they have spent in treatment. Although a patient's cocaine use generally stops at admission, the following measurable parameters should be used to determine when the next level of treatment should begin:

- level of drug craving
- level of psychological distress
- degree of resolution of the psychosocial crises that led to admission
- patients' knowledge and attitudes about recovery
- patients' support network

After discharge, a patient may experience intensified cravings, a relapse to drug use, or adverse change in his or her support network. These signs should signal a return to a more restrictive level of care. In some cases, this will mean returning to inpatient care.

Multiple Modality Treatment

Many stimulant abusers need both inpatient and residential care at some point in their recovery. Some stimulant abusers require inpatient psychiatric hospitalizations to contain toxic psychoses. Some may also require inpatient hospitalization to treat the medical complications of their stimulant abuse. Most, however, will need an initial phase of treatment in a chemical dependency center to interrupt their obsession with stimulant abuse and get started on a path to recovery.

Integration of Inpatient, Residential, and Outpatient Treatment

When treating a cocaine-dependent person, a clinician wants to know what kind of treatment will work best, given that person's particular circumstances. After the clinician determines what is needed, he or she wants to know how closely the ideal treatment situation can be approximated, given the real-life constraints that restrict the clinician's choice of options. For example, will the patient find the treatment acceptable? Can the patient afford the treatment either through insurance coverage, private payment, or availability of public funding?

Inpatient and outpatient benefits for medical insurance and disability often differ. Outpatient benefits are frequently more limited in scope and degree of reimbursement than are benefits for inpatient treatment, and the patient's share of the cost may be greater for outpatient even if the total cost of treatment is less. Because most patients suffering severe stimulant dependency are financially distressed, the patient's share of the cost is often an effective barrier to his or her obtaining treatment.

A similar situation often occurs with job disability and medical leave. When a patient is treated on an inpatient basis, disability insurance or medical leave is usually granted. The disability carrier or the patient's employer may assume, however, that a patient who can be treated as an outpatient is not "as sick" and may refuse to grant a job leave that is based on disability.

For optimal treatment of stimulant abusers, treatment staff would need to work with the same patient through inpatient or outpatient treatment and allow the patient to move from one level of care to another depending on progress, not time in treatment.

A stimulant-abusing patient might be treated as follows: If, at treatment entry, the patient was paranoid, out of behavioral control, and in need of behavioral containment, the patient would be best managed in an acute psychiatric hospital. After resolution of the acute psychosis, the patient would move to a chemical dependency recovery hospital that would provide a drug-free environment, introduction to the basics of recovery, and peer support for abstinence. When the patient had made a commitment to recovery and learned the basics of addiction and recovery, he or she would go to a halfway house or therapeutic community that would intensively support recovery twenty-four hours a day. Finally, the patient would return to live with his or her family.

Ideally, treatment would be conducted in comprehensive chemical dependency treatment centers where the flow from one treatment setting to another is not impeded by the staff's territorial or ideological boundaries, and where outpatient staff can continue working with a patient if rehospitalization should become necessary.

The best measures of treatment are not outcomes at some point in the future but are the ability to retain patients during the early stages of treatment, the patient's level of motivation, and the education of patients and their families about the process of recovery. The most important measure is the level of change in a patient's lifestyle orientation provided by the intensive intervention that often takes place in a treatment setting. Many members of AA call this change of lifestyle a "spiritual awakening."

Chapter 5
ENDNOTES

1. D. E. Smith and D. R. Wesson, *Uppers and Downers* (Englewood Cliffs, N. J.: Prentice-Hall, Inc., 1973).
2. D. E. Smith and D. R. Wesson, "Phenobarbital Technique for Treatment of Barbiturate Dependence," *Archives of General Psychiatry* 24 (1971): 56-60.
3. D. E. Smith, D. R. Wesson, and D. J. Tusel, *Treating Opiate Dependency* (Center City, Minn.: Hazelden Foundation, 1989).
4. A. M. Washton and Nannette Stone-Washton, "Abstinence and Relapse in Outpatient Cocaine Addicts," *Journal of Psychoactive Drugs* 22 (1990): 135-47; R. A. Rawson et al., "Neurobehavioral Treatment for Cocaine Dependency," *Journal of Psychoactive Drugs* 22 (1990): 159-71.

5. G. A. Marlatt, "Relapse Prevention: Theoretical Rationale and Overview of the Model," in *Relapse Prevention: Maintenance Strategies in the Treatment of Addictive Behaviors*, ed. G. A. Marlatt and J. R. Gordon (New York: Guilford, 1985).
6. M. O. Smith, "Acupuncture Treatment for Crack: Clinical Survey of 1,500 Patients Treated," *American Journal of Acupuncture* 16 (1988): 241-47.
7. D. Wyss, "A Hand and a Home for Pregnant Addicts," *Time* (27 February 1989): 10.
8. Jess G. Thoene, "Curing the Orphan Drug Act," *Science* 251 (1991): 1158-59.
9. F. H. Gawin and H. D. Kleber, "Cocaine Abuse Treatment: An Open Pilot Trial with Lithium and Desipramine," *Archives of General Psychiatry* 41 (1984): 903-10; T. R. Kosten et al., "A Preliminary Study of Desipramine in the Treatment of Cocaine Abuse in Methadone Maintenance Patients," *Journal of Clinical Psychiatry* 48 (1987): 442-44; F. H. Gawin et al., "Desipramine Facilitation of Initial Cocaine Abstinence," *Archives of General Psychiatry* 46 (1989): 117-21; M. W. Fishman and R. W. Foltin, "The Effects of Desipramine Maintenance on Cocaine Self-Administration in Humans," *Psychopharmacology* 96 (1998): S20.
10. C. A. Dackis, M. S. Gold, and A. L. C. Pottash, "Central Stimulant Abuse: Neurochemistry and Pharmacotherapy," *Advances in Alcohol and Substance Abuse* 6 (1987): 7-21.
11. L. Handelsman et al., "Amantadine for Treatment of Cocaine Dependence in Methadone-Maintained Patients," (letter) *American Journal of Psychiatry* 145 (1988): 533.
12. C. A. Dackis and M. S. Gold, "New Concepts in Cocaine Addiction: The Dopamine Depletion Hypothesis," *Neuroscience Biobehavioral Review* 9 (1985): 469-77; C. A. Dackis and M. S. Gold, "Bromocriptine as a Treatment of Cocaine Abuse," *Lancet* 1 (1985): 1151-52.
13. J. A. Corores et al., "Cocaine Abuse and Adult Attention Deficit Disorder," *Journal of Clinical Psychiatry* 48 (1987): 376-77.

14. N. K. Mell et al., "Buprenorphine Suppresses Cocaine Self-Administration by Rhesus Monkeys," *Science* 245 (1989): 859-62.

15. T. R. Kosten, H. D. Kleber, and C. Morgan, "Treatment of Cocaine Abuse with Buprenorphine," *Biological Psychiatry* 26 (1989): 637-39.

16. E. J. Khantzian, "An Extreme Case of Cocaine Dependence and Marked Improvement with Methylphenidate Treatment," *American Journal* 140 (1983): 784-85.

17. F. H. Gawin, C. Riodan, and H. D. Kleber, "Methylphenidate Treatment of Cocaine Abusers Without Attention Deficit Disorders: A Negative Report," *American Journal of Drug and Alcohol Abuse* 11 (1985): 193-97.

18. J. Halikas et al., "Carbamazepine for Cocaine Addiction," *Lancet* 1 (1989): 623-24.

19. F. H. Gawin, D. Allen, and B. Humblestone, "Outpatient Treatment of 'Crack' Cocaine Smoking with Flupentixol Decanoate," *Archives of General Psychiatry* 46 (1989): 322-25.

20. W. R. Miller and R. K. Hester, "Inpatient Alcoholism Treatment: Who Benefits?" *American Psychologist* 41 (1986): 794-805.

21. C. Holden, "Is Alcoholism Treatment Effective?" *Science* 236 (1987): 20-22.

6
PATHS TO ABSTINENCE

Stimulant addicts usually have no difficulty achieving brief periods of abstinence. The difficulty is not stopping but staying abstinent. When stimulant addicts are not using, they believe they are "in control" and that they can stay in control even if they use a small amount. Once loss of control has occurred, however, few who smoke stimulants ever reestablish it. Their only way of successfully coping with stimulants is complete, unremitting abstinence.

To achieve long-term abstinence, every addict must find a way that works for him or her. There is no one, or even best, path for every stimulant abuser. Counselors or psychotherapists can help addicts find the means of achieving long-term abstinence, but they must be able to tolerate the relapses that often occur before the goal of long-term abstinence is achieved.

From the addicts' perspective, abstinence from stimulants is easily achieved. They are sure that the next time they stop will be the last. Usually, they need to try their own methods until they exhaust themselves and eventually accept that they are incapable of staying quit on their own.

THE JOURNEY TO ABSTINENCE

The journey metaphor is a useful way to frame the steps an addict must go through before achieving long-term abstinence. As discussed in some detail in the introduction, metaphors and symbols are powerful ways of communicating. They reduce complex events to manageable terms and mold how we think and feel about something. The journey metaphor is simple and understood by everyone, yet it is powerful in working with addicts because it provides a rich terminology that minimizes fault (for example, a relapse becomes a wrong turn, a detour, losing one's way, or straying from the path). It defines the participants' roles—the addict is the one making the journey, the counselor is the guide—and provides an ultimate goal that doesn't have to be achieved all at once, but can be worked toward.

Addicts often perceive the need to stop or "cut back" their drug use before they believe it is possible to do so. They are ambivalent or unhappy about where they are in life, but see no options once they quit their drug use. The counselor's task is to allow the addict to see that continued drug use is not the inevitable result of genetics, psychopathology, environment, past deprivation or abuse, or prior drug use. Others have become abstinent and rebuilt their lives; therefore, so can they.

But there is also a trap. Counselors who are themselves recovering from alcohol or drug dependency generally have a strong emotional attachment to the method of abstinence that worked for them. Many counselors achieved their abstinence through a Twelve Step program and, understandably, want their clients to follow the same path. While Twelve Step recovery programs are an important path to achieving abstinence, they are not the only way. Insisting on Twelve Step work before the addict is ready for it can slow the recovery journey.

One must prepare for a journey. At minimum, one needs the best possible map. The counselor can provide education and anticipatory guidance about what is expected, how long the journey will take, how long it has taken others to make it, what pitfalls others have encountered, and what resources are available if the client gets off the path or makes a wrong turn.

Finally, one must embark on the journey, leaving behind what is familiar. Throughout the journey, the counselor is a guide, a touchstone, and a provider of support and encouragement. The journey is long, sometimes hard, and the way is not well marked. Mount Everest has been climbed many times and by different routes, but it is always climbed the same way: one step at a time. Endurance and methodical perseverance are more important than the ability to make big leaps.

GLOSSARY

BASEBALL. Freebase cocaine.

BATU. A street term for d-methamphetamine (a.k.a. ice).

BEAM ME UP, SCOTTY. A phrase from the TV series "Star Trek" that has become drug jargon for smoking cocaine freebase.

CAVIAR. Cocaine mixed in a tobacco cigarette. Originally referred to cocaine hydrochloride in a cigarette. Can also mean cocaine freebase in a cigarette.

CHASING AND BASING. Smoking heroin and cocaine together.

CHASING CASPER THE GHOST. Refers to smoking cocaine freebase.

CHASING THE DRAGON. Originally referred to smoking opium. More recently, it is also applied to smoking stimulants.

COCA PASTE. A crude extract of freebase that is smoked in South America.

CRANK. A street name for dl-methamphetamine crystals.

CRYSTAL. Can refer to d-methamphetamine (ice); dl-methamphetamine; or, on the East Coast, 4-methylaminorex (a.k.a. Euphoria or U4euH).

GRIMMIE. Crack cocaine added to a marijuana cigarette.

HEAD SHOPS. Stores that sell glass pipes, scales, and other drug use paraphernalia.

HUBBA. Crack cocaine.

ICE. Dextro-methamphetamine.

ICE CREAM. Another street term for ice.

L.A. GLASS. Another street term for ice.

NARCOTRAFICANTES. Cocaine traffickers in South America.

PRIMMIES. The combination of crack cocaine and a tobacco cigarette.

QUARTZ. Another street name for ice.

RICE. Another street name for ice.

SHABU. Another street name for d-methamphetamine (ice), used especially in the Philippines.

SHOWER POSSE. A violent Jamaican gang that controls much of the U.S. crack trade.

SPACEBASE. A mixture of cocaine and PCP that is smoked.

SPEED. Another street name for methamphetamine.

SPEEDBALL. A combination of heroin and cocaine, generally for injection.

TOSS-UP. A woman who trades sex for cocaine.

TWEAKING. "Seeing" cocaine on the floor, in the corner of one's visual field, causing users to sometimes get down on their hands and knees looking for the cocaine.

WHITE DOVE. Crack cocaine.

BOOKS AND OTHER REFERENCE MATERIALS

Chiang, C. N., and R. L. Hawks, eds. *Research Findings on Smoking of Abused Substances*. NIDA Research Monograph 99. Washington D.C.: U.S. Government Printing Office, 1990.

Clouet, D., K. Asghar, and R. Brown, eds. *Mechanism of Cocaine Abuse and Toxicity*. NIDA Research Monograph 88. Washingon, D.C.: Government Printing Office, 1988.

A technical review based on papers and discussions at a conference September 21-23, 1987, in Rockville, Md., sponsored by the Office of Science and the Division of Preclinical Research, NIDA. A highly technical presentation of interest primarily to preclinical scientists. The book is sold by the Superintendent of Documents, U.S. Government Printing Office, Washington, D.C. 20402.

Fisher, S., A. Raskin, and E. H. Uhlenhuth, eds. *Cocaine: Clinical and Behavioral Aspects*. Oxford, England: Oxford University Press, 1987.

Gold, M. S. *800-Cocaine*. Toronto, Canada: Bantam Books, 1984.

Harris, L. S. *Problems of Drug Dependence* 1987. NIDA Research Monograph 81. Washington, D.C.: U.S. Government Printing Office, 1988.

Jacobs, M. R., and K. Fehr. *Drugs and Drug Abuse: A Reference Text*. Toronto: Addiction Research Foundation, 1987. Reference with street terms.

Kozel, N. J., and E. H. Adams, eds. *Cocaine Use in America: Epidemiological and Clinical Perspectives*. NIDA Research Monograph 61. Washington, D.C.: U.S. Government Printing Office, 1985.

Miller, M. A., and N. J. Kozel, eds. *Methamphetamine Abuse: Epidemiological Issues and Implications*. NIDA Research Monograph 115. Washington, D.C.: U.S. Government Printing Office, 1991.

Thadani, P., ed. *Cardiovascular Toxicity of Cocaine: Underlying Mechanisms*. NIDA Research Monograph 108. Rockville, Md: U.S. Government Printing Office, 1991.

Turner, C. E., B. S. Urbanek, G. M. Wall, and C. W. Waller, *Cocaine: An Annotated Bibliography*. Jackson, Miss.: University Press of Mississippi, 1988.

This two volume set is an excellent guide to the cocaine literature before 1988. Volume 1 is the annotated bibliography. Volume 2 is the author and subject index.

Volkow, N. D., and A. C. Swann, eds. *Cocaine in the Brain*. New Brunswick, N. J.: Rutgers University Press, 1990.

Wallace, B. C. *Crack Cocaine: A Practical Treatment Approach for the Chemically Dependent*. New York: Brunner/Mazel, 1991.

Washton, A. M., and M. S. Gold, eds. *Cocaine: A Clinician's Handbook*. New York: Guilford Press, 1987.

INDEX

Carbamazepine, 70

"Caviar" (or "cavies"), 27

CDRH (Chemical dependency recovery hospitals). *See* Hospitals

"Chasing and basing," 27

"Chasing the dragon," 32

Chemical dependency recovery hospitals (CDRH). *See* Hospitals

Child abuse and neglect, 46

Classical conditioning, 60

Cocaine, 1-2, 5-7, 18, 19, 28; detection of, through urine testing, 34-35; forms of, 2, 21-23; medical complications of using, 39-48, 57, 77; methods of administering, 26-27; psychiatric complications of using, 51-53; treating addiction to, 4, 7-8, 55-81. *See also* Cocaine freebase; Crack cocaine

Cocaine alkaloid. *See* Cocaine freebase

Cocaine Anonymous, 58, 75

"Cocaine blues." *See* Withdrawal from drugs

Cocaine freebase, 2, 7, 21; as combined with other drugs, 27, 56; medical complications of using, 39-40; preparing, 22-23; street names for, 22, 23; subjective effects of using, 23-26. *See also* Cocaine; Crack cocaine

Cocaine hydrochloride. *See* Cocaine: Forms of

Coca paste, 1, 39

Counseling, 39, 53, 58; assistance of, in achieving abstinence, 85, 86; development of treatment plan in, 55-56; of minorities, 17-19

"Crack babies," 3, 44-47

Crack cocaine, 2-3, 10, 21, 53; and crime, 4-5; as combined with other drugs, 7, 27; as compared to methamphetamine, 9, 33; government response to epidemic of, 17-19; medical complications of using, 39-48; street names for, 23; subjective effects of using, 23-26; treating addiction to, 4, 58-59, 62. *See also* Cocaine; Cocaine freebase; "Crack babies"

"Crack lung," 41

"Crank." *See* Methamphetamine: Street names for

"Crash." *See* Withdrawal from drugs

Cravings: for cocaine, 25, 28, 61, 79; for ice, 33; reducing through medication, 40, 68, 69, 70; relapses caused by, 60, 67

Crime, 5

"Crystal." *See* 4-methylaminorex; Ice: Other street names for

D

DEA. *See* Drug Enforcement Administration

Hispanics, 3, 8, 18
HIV infection, 26-27, 42, 43. *See also* AIDS
HMOs. *See* Health maintenance organizations
Hospitals: chemical dependency recovery, 75, 76, 78, 80, 81; medical, 77; psychiatric, 77-78. *See also* Treatment of drug abuse: Inpatient vs. outpatient
"Hubba." *See* Crack cocaine: Street names for

I

Ice, 9-10, 30; medical complications of using, 39, 47; other street names for, 10, 31; subjective effects of using, 33-34. *See also* Methamphetamine
"Ice babies," 47
"Ice cream." *See* Ice: Other street names for
Imipramine, 53
Infections. *See* Hepatitis; HIV infection; Tuberculosis
Injecting drugs. *See* Intravenous injection of drugs
Inpatient treatment. *See* Treatment of drug abuse: Inpatient vs. outpatient
Intravenous injection of drugs, 7, 26-27, 32, 39

J

Jobs. *See* Workplace

L

"L.A. glass." *See* Ice: Other street names for
Levo-methamphetamine. *See* Methamphetamine: Structure and forms of

M

MAMA Project. *See* Moving Addicted Mothers Ahead
Managed health care, 72-73
Mandela House, 62-63
Marijuana, 2, 41; as combined with other drugs, 10, 27, 33
Media: role of, in drug abuse, 5-7, 9-10
Medical insurance, 7, 8, 16, 56, 72, 73, 74, 80
Medical model of drug abuse treatment, 14-17
Methadone, 12, 68, 69, 70
Methamphetamine, 1, 56; detection of, through urine testing, 34-35, 36; medical complications of using, 39-48, 57, 77; methods of administering, 32-33; psychiatric complications of using, 51-53; street names for, 9, 31; structure and forms of, 28-32; treating addiction to, 55-81. *See also* Ice
Methamphetamine freebase. *See* Methamphetamine: Structure and forms of
Methedrine, 8
Methylphenidate, 68, 70

Minorities. *See* Blacks; Hispanics

Moving Addicted Mothers Ahead, 63

Multiple modality treatment, 79

Myocardial infarction, 42, 77

N

Naltrexone, 68

National Institute on Drug Abuse (NIDA), 3, 47-48, 63-65

Neurotransmitters, 44, 66, 69

NIDA. *See* National Institute on Drug Abuse

Norepinephrine. *See* Neurotransmitters.

O

Opiates, 6, 56-57, 68-70. *See also* Heroin

Orphan Drug Act of 1983, 64

Outpatient treatment. *See* Treatment of drug abuse: Inpatient vs. outpatient

P

Panic attacks. *See* Anxiety disorders

Paranoia, 5, 9, 26, 52, 80

Paranoid schizophrenia. *See* Schizophrenia

Pavlovian conditioning. *See* Classical conditioning

PCP, 31

PDE toddler. *See* Prenatal drug-exposed toddler

Peruvian Indians, drug use among, 1

Pharmaceutical companies, 63-64

Pharmaceutical Manufacturer's Association, 63

Phenylpropanolamine, 36

Philippines, ice abuse in, 9, 10, 47

Pneumomediastinum, 41-42

Pregnant drug abusers: and "crack babies," 44-47; and "ice babies," 47; treating, 62-63

Prenatal drug-exposed toddler, 45-46

"Primmies," 27

Psychopathology, 51-53, 67-71

Psychosis. *See* Schizophrenia; Stimulant psychosis

Psychotherapy, 16, 59-60

Q

"Quartz." *See* Ice: Other street names for

R

Racism, 18

Recovery groups, 8, 15, 57. *See also* Twelve Step recovery

Relapse, 51, 57, 60, 79; preventing, through medication, 65, 67-68

"Rice." *See* Ice: Other street names for

"Rock," *See* Cocaine freebase: Street names for

S

Schizophrenia, 12, 51-52

Sedative-hypnotics, 57

Other titles for your professional development . . .

Outpatient Treatment of Cocaine and Crack Addiction
Making It Work
by Dr. Arnold M. Washton and Nannette Stone-Washton
With increasing pressure to contain treatment costs, numerous
treatment providers are turning to outpatient treatment services.
This pamphlet, while focusing on outpatient treatment of cocaine
and crack addiction, also offers suggestions for creating outpatient
programs that work in the treatment of other chemical addictions.
Pamphlet, 10 pp.
Order No. 5189

Treating Opiate Dependency
*by David E. Smith, M.D., Donald R. Wesson, M.D., and
Donald J. Tusel, M.D.*
Filled with extensive clinical experience and research knowledge,
Treating Opiate Dependency is one of the most valuable reference
books for professionals today. You'll learn proven assessment and
treatment techniques for working with opiate-addicted clients. A
thorough overview of methadone maintenance programs is con-
trasted with traditional drug-free treatment. Paperback, 113 pp.
Order No. 5164

The New Drugs
Look-Alikes, Drugs of Deception, and Designer Drugs
*by Richard Seymour, M.A., David Smith, M.D., Darryl Inaba,
Pharm.D., and Mim Landry*
The New Drugs is a concise survey of the four major categories
of psychoactive drugs available today. You'll discover the impact
drug enforcement, research, and legislation can have on new drugs.
Essential identification, assessment, and treatment guidelines are
outlined to assist a wide range of health care professionals.
Paperback, 164 pp.
Order No. 5054

**For price and order information, or a free catalog,
please call our Telephone Representatives.**

HAZELDEN EDUCATIONAL MATERIALS

1-800-328-9000   **1-612-257-4010**   **1-612-257-1331**
(Toll Free. U.S., Canada,   (Outside the U.S. & Canada)   (FAX)
& the Virgin Islands)

15251 Pleasant Valley Road • P.O. Box 176 • Center City, MN 55012-0176
Hazelden Europe
P.O. Box 616
Cork, Ireland
Phone: Int'l. Code+353+21+314318
24-Hour FAX: Int'l. Code+353+21+961269